Performance Ch
for Lammon, Fc

CLINICAL NURSING SKILLS

PEGGY A. ELLIS, PhD, RN
BARBARA R. HARBIN, MS, RN, CCRN

School of Nursing
University of Alabama at Birmingham
Birmingham, Alabama

W.B. SAUNDERS COMPANY

A Division of Harcourt Brace & Company
Philadelphia   London   Toronto   Montreal

D1638859

W.B. SAUNDERS COMP
A Division of Harcourt Br

The Curtis Center
Independence Square Wes
Philadelphia, Pennsylvani

Performance Checklists for Lammon, Foote, Leli, Ingle, and Adams: Clinical Nursing Skills   ISBN 0-7216-5848-2

Printed in the United States of America.

Last digit is the print number: 9   8   7   6   5   4   3   2   1

PREFACE

Self-evaluation and feedback from others are necessary components of learning a new skill. These *Performance Checklists for Lammon, Foote, Leli, Ingle, and Adams: Clinical Nursing Skills* were designed to help you evaluate how well you have learned to perform the various skills necessary to the art and science of nursing. Each checklist corresponds to a skill in *Clinical Nursing Skills* by Carol Barnett Lammon, Anne W. Foote, Patricia G. Leli, Janice Ingle, and Marsha H. Adams.

You can use these checklists in several ways:

- To review the critical steps of a particular skill;
- As a self-evaluation exercise after performing a particular skill;
- In conjunction with your instructor, who can use the forms to give you specific feedback on your performance. Each checklist includes spaces in which your instructor can evaluate your performance of each step as satisfactory ("S") or unsatisfactory ("U"), as well as spaces for comments.

The Table of Contents will help you quickly locate the checklist you need. In addition, the checklist numbers correspond to the skill numbers in *Clinical Nursing Skills.* The pages are perforated for easy removal of individual checklists.

It is hoped that these checklists, in conjunction with *Clinical Nursing Skills,* will help you learn, practice, and perfect the diverse skills necessary to the safe, efficient, and effective care of your patients.

CONTENTS

Contents

Contents

Contents

Name _____   Specific Skill Performed _____
Date _____   Attempt Number _____
Instructor _____   PASS _____   FAIL _____

PERFORMANCE CHECKLIST 1.1   HANDWASHING

		S	U	COMMENTS
1.	Removed rings and jewelry.			
2.	Adjusted water temperature to comfortable level using a paper towel to turn on the water.			
3.	Wet hands well and applied 1 tablespoon of soap while avoiding splashing of water and holding hands lower than elbows.			
4.	Rubbed all aspects of palms and fingers together using friction for at least 10 seconds.			
5.	Cleaned under fingernails with small brush.			
6.	Rinsed hands under running water, keeping fingers lower than wrists.			
7.	Dried hands with paper towel wiping from fingertips to wrist.			
8.	Turned off water using another paper towel.			
9.	Discarded paper towels correctly.			

Additional Comments:

_____

_____

_____

_____

_____

_____

_____

_____

_____

_____

Name _____

Date _____

Instructor _____

Specific Skill Performed _____

Attempt Number _____

PASS _____   FAIL _____

PERFORMANCE CHECKLIST 1.2   **DONNING AND REMOVING A PROTECTIVE GOWN**

	S	U	COMMENTS
1. Assessed medical diagnosis and need for gown.			
2. Washed hands.			
3. Picked up gown and allowed it to unfold without touching the floor.			
4. Held inside of gown in front of you.			
5. Put on gown with opening in back.			
6. Tied gown at neck making sure gown overlaps in back.			
7. Tied gown at waist.			
Removing the Gown			
8. Untied the Gown.			
9. Removed gown, folding it inside out as you remove it.			
10. Placed gown in appropriate receptacle.			
11. Removed gloves, if necessary.			
12. Washed hands.			
13. Documented precautions used.			

Additional Comments:

_____

_____

_____

_____

_____

_____

_____

_____

Name _____

Date _____

Instructor _____

PERFORMANCE CHECKLIST 1.3   DONNING AND REMOVING A PROTECTIVE FACE MASK AND EYEWEAR

	S	U	COMMENTS
1. Reviewed medical diagnosis and need for mask and eyewear.			
2. Washed hands.			
3. Explained to client need for eyewear and mask.			
4. Put on eye protection.			
5. Grasped mask by strings without touching the middle part of mask.			
6. Molded metal piece to bridge of nose.			
7. Tied top strings around head at occipital area.			
8. Tied lower strings around neck.			
9. Left no gaps around edges of mask.			
To Remove			
10. Untied lower two strings of mask first and then upper strings.			
11. Held top string while bringing mask away from face.			
12. Disposed of mask in the appropriate receptacle.			
13. Washed hands.			
14. Documented precautions used.			

Additional Comments:

_____

_____

_____

_____

_____

_____

Name _____   Specific Skill Performed _____

Date _____   Attempt Number _____

Instructor _____   PASS _____   FAIL _____

PERFORMANCE CHECKLIST 1.4   DONNING AND REMOVING DISPOSABLE EXAMINATION GLOVES

	S	U	COMMENTS
1. Reviewed medical diagnosis and need for gloves.			
2. Washed hands.			
3. Slipped hands into gloves.			
Removing Soiled Gloves			
4. Used nondominant hand to grasp outside cuff of other glove.			
5. Removed glove by turning it inside out as you pulled it off.			
6. Holding the just-removed glove in gloved hand, slid ungloved fingers under cuff of soiled glove and pulled glove off turning it inside out over glove you continue to hold.			
7. Discarded gloves in appropriate receptacle.			

Additional Comments:

_____

_____

_____

_____

_____

_____

_____

_____

_____

_____

_____

PERFORMANCE CHECKLIST 1.5   **DONNING AND REMOVING SHOE COVERS, CAP, AND SURGICAL MASK**

	S	U	COMMENTS
1. Reviewed medical diagnosis and need for shoe covers, cap, and surgical mask.			
2. Washed hands. Secured hair away from face if necessary.			
3. Put on shoe covers correctly.			
4. Placed cap on head so that all hair is covered.			
5. Picked up mask by strings.			
6. Followed steps 6-9 in Performance Checklist 1.3.			
Removing Cap, Mask, and Shoe Covers			
7. Removed gown and gloves before removing mask.			
8. Untied lower strings of mask then upper strings.			
9. Discarded mask touching only the strings.			
10. Removed cap and discarded in appropriate receptacle.			
11. Removed shoe covers and discarded in appropriate receptacle.			
12. Documented precautions used.			

Additional Comments:

_____

_____

_____

_____

_____

_____

_____

Name _____ Specific Skill Performed _____

Date _____ Attempt Number _____

Instructor _____ PASS _____ FAIL _____

PERFORMANCE CHECKLIST 1.6   **PERFORMING A SURGICAL HAND SCRUB**

	S	U	COMMENTS
1. Put on proper surgical attire including mask, and removed all jewelry.			
2. Obtained brush and placed open package near sink.			
3. Adjusted water temperature to comfortable level.			
4. Avoided touching sink with hands or clothes.			
5. Wet hands and forearms while keeping hands and forearms above elbows and away from clothing.			
6. Applied 1 teaspoon of antimicrobial soap and lathered hands and forearms.			
7. Used fingernail cleaner to clean under each fingernail on each hand and discarded fingernail cleaner.			
8. Scrubbed each surface of each hand using sponge side of brush and then bristle side of brush beginning with fingernails and progressing to wrists according to timed or counted stroke method.			
9. Scrubbed each surface of each forearm with sponge side of brush and then bristle side of brush beginning at wrists and progressing to within 10 cm. of elbow.			
10. Discarded scrub brush and fully rinsed each arm under running water beginning with fingertips and moving to elbow.			
11. Kept fingers and hands higher than elbows without touching any surface.			
12. Turned off water without contaminating hands.			
13. Dried each hand and arm with sterile towel working from fingertips to elbows.			
14. Discarded towels in appropriate receptacle.			
15. Kept hands above waist and in line of vision.			

Additional Comments:

_____

_____

Name _____   Specific Skill Performed _____
Date _____   Attempt Number _____
Instructor _____   PASS _____   FAIL _____

PERFORMANCE CHECKLIST 1.7   DONNING AND REMOVING A STERILE GOWN

	S	U	COMMENTS
1. Washed hands.			
2. Checked sterile package for signs of contamination.			
3. Placed gown package waist-high on clean, flat, dry surface.			
4. Put on hair cover and mask, if indicated.			
5. Completed surgical scrub of hands.			
6. Opened outer wrapper of gown correctly.			
7. Picked up gown by inside of neck touching only the side of the gown which will be next to you.			
8. Lifted gown up and away from sterile field while stepping back.			
9. Held gown with upper half in front of you and allowed gown to unfold away from other objects.			
10. Worked arms into sleeve openings while raising and spreading arms.			
11. Kept hands within sleeves while assistant adjusted sleeves from inside and tied gown.			
12. Put on gloves (see Performance Checklist 1.8).			
Removing the Soiled Gown			
13. Untied strings of gown.			
14. Removed gown folding it inside out to cover outside of gown.			
15. Discarded gown in appropriate receptacle.			
16. Removed gloves (see Performance Checklist 1.8).			
17. Washed hands.			
18. Documented precautions used.			

Name _____   Specific Skill Performed _____

Date _____   Attempt Number _____

Instructor _____   PASS _____   FAIL _____

PERFORMANCE CHECKLIST 1.8 DONNING AND REMOVING STERILE GLOVES

	S	U	COMMENTS
1. Reviewed medical diagnosis and need for sterile gloves.			
2. Washed hands thoroughly.			
3. Placed unopened package of gloves on clean, dry surface.			
4. Opened outside paper covering sterile gloves correctly.			
5. Removed outer wrapper. Laid exposed package of gloves on clean, dry surface with cuff end of gloves toward you.			
6. Opened inner package touching only the bottom of the package.			
7. Using thumb and finger of nondominant hand, grasped cuff portion of glove for dominant hand and lifted glove while holding fingers down.			
8. Carefully slipped hand inside glove with thumb and fingers in proper spaces and without contaminating glove.			
9. Using gloved hand, slid fingers under cuffed portion of other glove.			
10. Slid second glove on hand with thumb and fingers in proper spaces and without contaminating glove.			
11. Adjusted gloves for proper fit with cuffs up without touching nonsterile surface.			
Removing the Soiled Gloves			
12. Grasped outside cuff of one glove and pulled it off inside out.			
13. Slid fingers under cuff of remaining gloved hand and removed glove inside out.			
14. Disposed of gloves in proper receptacle.			
15. Documented precautions used.			

Additional Comments:

_____

_____

Name _____   Specific Skill Performed _____
Date _____   Attempt Number _____
Instructor _____   PASS _____   FAIL _____

PERFORMANCE CHECKLIST 1.9   PREPARING AND MAINTAINING A STERILE FIELD

	S	U	COMMENTS
1. Reviewed medical diagnosis and need for sterile field.			
2. Inspected wrapping around sterile packaging for signs of contamination.			
3. Washed hands.			
4. Set up sterile field on waist-high table.			
Setting up a Prepackaged Sterile Tray			
5. Removed tape and folded back first flap away from you.			
6. Using both hands, pulled two middle flaps open.			
7. Pulled remaining flap toward you, exposing sterile tray.			
Adding Wrapped Items to a Sterile Field			
8. Held sterile package securely while unwrapping.			
9. Folded back first flap away from you while still holding the package.			
10. Correctly folded back side flaps, one at a time.			
11. Unfolded last flap toward you exposing item.			
12. Held wrapper out of the way of the sterile field while dropping sterile item onto sterile field inside 1-inch border.			
Pouring a Solution into a Sterile Basin			
13. Made sure a sterile container for antiseptic solution is present on tray inside 1-inch border.			
14. Held antiseptic solution with label on top.			
15. Held bottle above tray and carefully poured solution into sterile container without splashing or spilling solution.			

	S	U	COMMENTS
Adding Prepackaged Items to a Sterile Field			
16. Opened package correctly without contaminating the contents.			
17. Dropped item onto sterile field inside 1-inch border.			
Preparing a Sterile Field Using a Disposable Drape			
18. Correctly opened sterile package containing drape without contaminating drape.			
19. Removed sterile drape by the corner and allowed it to unfold.			
20. Placed sterile drape on table from back to front without contaminating.			
21. Placed sterile items within the sterile field correctly.			
22. If forceps were stored in disinfectant solution, held them with tips lower than your wrist.			
23. Did not allow forceps to touch nonsterile objects.			
24. Grasped sterile items with forceps and transferred to sterile field without contamination.			

Additional Comments:

_____

_____

_____

_____

_____

_____

_____

_____

_____

_____

Name _____   Specific Skill Performed _____

Date _____   Attempt Number _____

Instructor _____   PASS _____   FAIL _____

PERFORMANCE CHECKLIST 2.1   GENERAL PRINCIPLES OF BODY MECHANICS

	S	U	COMMENTS
1. Assessed need for help and obtained help if necessary.			
2. Stood with feet apart and firm.			
3. Kept center of gravity low and centered over base of support.			
4. Lifted object from floor using leg and hip muscles and keeping back straight.			
5. Used smooth, coordinated movements to lift and move an object.			
6. Maintained good spinal alignment.			
7. Pushed, pulled or slid an object instead of lifting when possible.			
8. Held load close to body when carrying.			
9. Used entire hand instead of fingers. Used arms as levers.			
10. Used "internal girdle" to protect lower intervertebral discs.			

Additional Comments:

_____

_____

_____

_____

_____

_____

_____

_____

_____

_____

Name _____   Specific Skill Performed _____
Date _____   Attempt Number _____
Instructor _____   PASS _____   FAIL _____

PERFORMANCE CHECKLIST 3.1   **PERFORMING CARDIOPULMONARY RESUSCITATION**

	S	U	COMMENTS
PERFORMING ONE-PERSON CPR			
1. Assessed victim for unresponsiveness. Determined need for CPR.			
2. Called for help per agency policy. Activated EMS if outside hospital.			
3. Placed victim in rescue position (horizontal, supine on firm flat surface).			
Airway			
4. Used appropriate technique to open victim's airway (head tilt/ chin lift or jaw thrust if neck injury suspected).			
5. Determined breathlessness (look, listen, feel for 5 to 10 seconds).			
Breathing			
6. If respirations present, maintained airway and monitored breathing.			
7. If respirations absent, used appropriate technique to initiate artificial ventilation (mouth to mouth, mouth to stoma, mouth to barrier device, bag-valve-mask device).			
8. Gave 2 slow breaths initially (1.5 to 2 seconds each) and allowed for exhalation.			
9. Repositioned victim and re-attempted ventilation if unsuccessful initially.			
10. If airway obstructed, used appropriate technique to remove obstruction (see Performance Checklist 3.3).			
Circulation			
11. Assessed for presence of major pulse after initial ventilation (carotid if adult or child, brachial if infant). Palpated pulse for minimum of 5 seconds but no longer than 10 seconds.			

	S	U	COMMENTS
12. If pulse present but victim breathless, continued rescue breathing at proper rate per minute (adult 10 to 12, child 15, infant 20) until spontaneous respirations begin.			
13. If pulse absent, positioned self to perform cardiac compressions.			
14. Used appropriate technique to locate proper hand placement on victim's chest.			
15. Performed chest compressions at proper depth and rate.			
16. Interposed artificial ventilation at proper rate and time during CPR.			
17. After one minute of CPR, reassessed victim for spontaneous respiration and return of pulse. Did not interrupt CPR for more than 5 seconds.			
18. Resumed CPR if victim still unresponsive.			
19. Periodically assessed victim's cardiopulmonary status.			
Continuation/Termination of CPR			
20. Continued CPR as necessary until: a. effective respirations and circulation returned b. relieved by other rescuers or CPR team c. termination by decision that it was futile d. rescuer exhaustion			
21. Appropriately reported/documented circumstances of victim cardiopulmonary arrest and resuscitation activities.			

Additional Comments:

_____

_____

_____

_____

_____

_____

_____

_____

	S	U	COMMENTS
PERFORMING TWO-PERSON CPR			
1. Assessed victim for unresponsiveness. Determined need for CPR.			
2. Called for help per agency policy. Activated EMS if outside hospital.			
3. Placed victim in rescue position (horizontal, supine on firm flat surface).			
Airway			
4. Used appropriate technique to open victim's airway (head tilt/ chin lift or jaw thrust if neck injury suspected).			
5. Determined breathlessness (look, listen, feel for 5 to 10 seconds).			
Breathing			
6. If respirations present, maintained airway and monitored breathing.			
7. If respirations absent, used appropriate technique to initiate artificial ventilation (mouth to mouth, mouth to stoma, mouth to barrier device, bag-valve-mask device).			
8. Gave 2 slow breaths initially (1.5 to 2 seconds each) and allowed for exhalation.			
9. Repositioned victim and re-attempted ventilation if unsuccessful initially.			
10. If airway obstructed, used appropriate technique to remove obstruction (see Performance Checklist 3.3).			
Circulation			
11. First rescuer assessed for presence of major pulse after giving initial ventilation. Palpated pulse for minimum of 5 seconds but no longer than 10 seconds.			
12. If pulse present but victim breathless, second rescuer began artificial ventilation at proper rate until spontaneous respirations began.			

	S	U	COMMENTS
13. If pulse absent, first rescuer positioned self at level of victim's chest on opposite side from second rescuer and prepared to perform cardiac compressions.			
14. First rescuer used appropriate technique to locate proper hand placement on victim's chest.			
15. First rescuer performed chest compression at proper depth and rate. Used mnemonic to aid with timing/coordinate efforts of both rescuers.			
16. Second rescuer interposed artificial ventilation at proper rate and time in coordination with first rescuer.			
17. After one minute of CPR, first rescuer reassessed victim for spontaneous respiration and return of pulse. Did not interrupt CPR for more than 5 seconds.			
18. Resumed CPR if victim still unresponsive.			
19. First rescuer periodically assessed victim's cardiopulmonary status.			
Change of Rescuer Role			
20. When fatigued, the compressor (first rescuer) signaled the need for relief.			
21. The second rescuer delivered one ventilation and moved to the victim's chest.			
22. While the first rescuer moved to the victim's head, delivered one breath and assessed for the presence of a pulse, the second rescuer located proper hand placement for chest compression.			
23. If victim remained pulseless, the first rescuer signaled for compressions to resume.			
Continuation/Termination of CPR			
24. Continued CPR as necessary until: a. effective respirations and circulation returned b. relieved by other rescuers or CPR team c. termination by decision that it was futile d. rescuer exhaustion			
25. Appropriately reported/documented circumstances of victim cardiopulmonary arrest and resuscitation activities.			

Name _____   Specific Skill Performed _____

Date _____   Attempt Number _____

Instructor _____   PASS _____   FAIL _____

PERFORMANCE CHECKLIST 3.2   USING A BAG-VALVE-MASK DEVICE (AMBU BAG)

	S	U	COMMENTS
1. Assessed client's condition and airway patency. Determined need for ambu bag.			
2. Obtained necessary equipment and prepared it for use. Turned on oxygen if appropriate.			
3. Washed hands if time permits.			
4. Used appropriate technique to open airway. Inserted oral airway if needed (see Performance Checklist 17.9).			
5. Used one hand to maintain head in open airway position. Placed mask firmly over client's nose and mouth with other hand (or attached adapter to artificial airway tube if client intubated).			
6. Used fingers of first hand to hold mask firmly in place while maintaining open airway with heel of hand.			
7. Used free hand to compress and release the bag reservoir in a slow, rhythmical motion at a rate of 12 to 20 times per minute.			
8. Coordinated ventilation with chest compressions if CPR performed (see Performance Checklist for 2 person CPR).			
9. Observed for chest rise and fall. Observed for gastric distention.			
10. Periodically assessed client for return of spontaneous respirations.			
11. Appropriately reported/documented procedure, client condition and assessment data.			

Additional Comments:

_____

_____

_____

_____

_____

_____

Name _____   Specific Skill Performed _____
Date _____   Attempt Number _____
Instructor _____   PASS _____   FAIL _____

PERFORMANCE CHECKLIST 3.3   **MANAGING A FOREIGN BODY AIRWAY OBSTRUCTION**

	S	U	COMMENTS
MANAGING THE CONSCIOUS VICTIM			
1. If choking suspected, quickly assessed victim and determined if foreign body airway obstruction complete or partial (i.e., asked "Can you speak?"). Called for help.			
2. If obstruction partial (i.e., victim able to speak and cough), encouraged strong forceful coughing to relieve obstruction. Remained with victim.			
3. If obstruction complete (i.e., victim unable to speak, cough or breathe) attempted to remove obstruction.			
Adult or Child Over 1 Year			
4. Applied 5 manual abdominal thrusts (or 5 chest thrusts if victim obese or pregnant).			
5. Repeated manual thrusts until obstruction cleared or victim becomes unconscious.			
Infant			
6. Properly placed infant over rescuer arm in head-low, face-down position and administered 5 back blows.			
7. Turned infant over and gave 5 chest thrusts.			
8. Opened infant's mouth and inspected oral cavity for foreign body. If visible, removed it with fingers and attempted ventilation.			
9. Repeated steps 6-8 until obstruction cleared and ventilation established.			

	S	U	COMMENTS
MANAGING THE CONSCIOUS VICTIM WHO BECOMES UNCONSCIOUS			
10. Activated EMS (if not already done).			
11. Placed victim in rescue position and used appropriate technique to open airway.			
12. Attempted to ventilate victim. Assessed for ventilation effectiveness (i.e., look, listen, feel).			
13. If unable to ventilate, attempted to remove obstruction.			
Adult or Child Over 1 Year			
14. Positioned self astride victim's thighs and administered 5 manual abdominal thrusts (or 5 chest thrusts if appropriate).			
15. Opened victim's mouth and inspected oral cavity for foreign body. If visible (epiglottis or above), performed finger sweep (with gloves if available).			
16. Reposition victim's head and attempted ventilation.			
17. Repeated steps 14-16 until obstruction cleared and ventilation established.			
MANAGING THE UNCONSCIOUS VICTIM (UNDETERMINED CAUSE)			
18. Determined unresponsiveness.			
19. Activated EMS.			
20. Placed victim in rescue position, opened airway and assessed for respirations.			
21. If no respirations present, attempted to ventilate victim. Repositioned head and attempted again to ventilate if unsuccessful on first try.			
22. If unable to ventilate, followed steps 14-17 until obstruction cleared and ventilation established.			

Additional Comments:

_____

_____

Name _____   Specific Skill Performed _____

Date _____   Attempt Number _____

Instructor _____   PASS _____   FAIL _____

PERFORMANCE CHECKLIST 4.1   MEASURING TYMPANIC TEMPERATURE

	S	U	COMMENTS
1. Assessed temperature readings over last 24 hours and medical diagnosis.			
2. Washed hands and explained procedure to client.			
3. Removed probe from base unit and noted lighted display.			
4. Checked that machine is in tympanic mode.			
5. Placed disposable cover on probe tip.			
6. Pressed scan button while inserting probe tip into and sealing client's ear canal.			
7. Released scan button.			
8. Removed probe when signaled that thermometer has registered.			
9. Read and recorded temperature correctly.			
10. Discarded probe cover into waste receptacle.			
11. Returned probe to charger.			
12. Washed hands.			
13. Assessed results and explained to client. Notified appropriate personnel.			
14. Documented results correctly.			

Additional Comments:

_____

_____

_____

_____

_____

_____

_____

Name _____   Specific Skill Performed _____

Date _____   Attempt Number _____

Instructor _____   PASS _____   FAIL _____

PERFORMANCE CHECKLIST 4.2   **MEASURING ORAL TEMPERATURE**

	S	U	COMMENTS
1. Assessed temperature readings over last 24 hours and medical diagnosis.			
2. Washed hands and explained procedure to client.			
Using a Glass Thermometer			
3. Held thermometer at end opposite bulb and rinsed in cold water.			
4. Correctly dried thermometer with tissue and shook down mercury.			
5. Inserted thermometer into sheath and removed paper.			
6. Placed thermometer in client's posterior sublingual pocket and instructed client to keep mouth closed.			
7. Left thermometer in place an appropriate length of time and removed from client's mouth.			
8. Removed sheath and read thermometer correctly. If sheath not used, cleaned thermometer correctly and returned to disinfectant solution.			
9. Recorded temperature correctly.			
Using an Electronic Thermometer			
10. Removed thermometer from charger and made sure blue probe was attached.			
11. Placed probe cover on probe and placed in client's posterior sublingual pocket. Instructed client to keep lips closed around probe.			
12. Read results from display when machine emitted a tone.			
13. Discarded probe cover and replaced thermometer on charger.			
14. Washed hands.			
15. Assessed results and explained to client. Reported to appropriate personnel.			
16. Documented results correctly.			

Name _____   Specific Skill Performed _____
Date _____   Attempt Number _____
Instructor _____   PASS _____   FAIL _____

PERFORMANCE CHECKLIST 4.3   **MEASURING RECTAL TEMPERATURE**

	S	U	COMMENTS
1. Assessed temperature readings over last 24 hours and medical diagnosis.			
2. Explained procedure to client.			
Using a Glass Thermometer			
3. Held thermometer at end opposite the bulb and rinsed in cold water. Dried correctly.			
4. Provided for client privacy and positioned client correctly.			
5. Applied gloves.			
6. Shook down thermometer and placed in sheath correctly or lubricated bulb with water-soluble jelly.			
7. Spread the client's buttocks and inserted thermometer into anus correctly.			
8. Held thermometer in place for appropriate length of time.			
9. Removed the thermometer. Pulled off sheath or removed secretions wiping from stem to bulb.			
10. Read thermometer correctly.			
11. Clean thermometer properly with soap and water.			
Using an Electronic Thermometer			
12. Removed thermometer from charger and attached red probe.			
13. Placed probe cover on probe and lubricated tip with water-soluble jelly.			
14. Protected client's privacy and positioned client correctly.			
15. Spread client's buttocks and inserted probe correctly.			
16. Remained with client and held probe in place.			

	S	U	COMMENTS
17. Read results from display when machine emitted a tone.			
18. Discarded probe cover and replaced thermometer on charger.			
19. Washed hands.			
20. Assessed results and explained to client. Reported to appropriate personnel.			
21. Documented results correctly.			

Additional Comments:

_____

_____

_____

_____

_____

_____

_____

_____

_____

_____

_____

_____

_____

_____

Name _____

Date _____

Instructor _____

Specific Skill Performed _____

Attempt Number _____

PASS _____   FAIL _____

PERFORMANCE CHECKLIST 4.4   **MEASURING AXILLARY TEMPERATURE**

	S	U	COMMENTS
1. Assessed temperature readings over last 24 hours and medical diagnosis.			
2. Explained procedure to client.			
Using a Glass Thermometer			
3. Held thermometer at end opposite the bulb and rinsed in cold water. Dried correctly.			
4. Shook down thermometer correctly.			
5. Positioned client to allow access to axillary area.			
6. Placed bulb of thermometer in client's axilla. Instructed client to hold arm firmly against the thorax.			
7. Left thermometer in place for 5 to 7 minutes and removed from axilla.			
8. Read thermometer correctly.			
9. Cleaned thermometer correctly using soap and water. Returned to disinfectant solution.			
Using an Electronic Thermometer			
10. Follow steps 14 and 15 from Performance Checklist 4.2.			
11. Placed covered probe in client's axilla with client's arm held firmly against thorax.			
12. When machine emits tone, read digital display correctly.			
13. Followed steps 18 through 21 from Performance Checklist 4.2.			

Additional Comments:

_____

_____

_____

Name _____   Specific Skill Performed _____
Date _____   Attempt Number _____
Instructor _____   PASS _____   FAIL _____

PERFORMANCE CHECKLIST 4.5   MEASURING RADIAL PULSE

	S	U	COMMENTS
1. Assessed previous pulse rates obtained and medical diagnosis.			
2. Assessed if client is taking medications which may affect pulse rate.			
3. Explained procedure to client.			
4. Placed client in position of comfort and located client's radial pulse.			
5. Palpated pulse correctly. Determined if pulse is regular and the rate. Also noted rhythm and volume of pulse.			
6. Assessed results and explained to client if appropriate. Notified appropriate personnel.			
7. Washed hands.			
8. Documented correctly.			

Additional Comments:

_____

_____

_____

_____

_____

_____

_____

_____

_____

_____

_____

_____

Name _____   Specific Skill Performed _____
Date _____   Attempt Number _____
Instructor _____   PASS _____   FAIL _____

PERFORMANCE CHECKLIST 4.6   MEASURING APICAL PULSE

	S	U	COMMENTS
1. Assessed previous pulse rate readings and medical diagnosis.			
2. Determined medications client is taking which may affect pulse rate.			
3. Explained procedure to client.			
4. Washed hands. Placed client in position of comfort and located apical area of heart.			
5. Cleansed stethoscope properly. Warmed endpiece of stethoscope.			
6. Placed eartips of stethoscope in ears correctly and diaphragm of stethoscope over apical area of chest.			
7. Counted heart rate for 1 minute, noting rhythm.			
8. Assessed results and explained to client if appropriate. Reported to appropriate personnel.			
9. Washed hands.			
10. Documented results correctly.			

Additional Comments:

_____

_____

_____

_____

_____

_____

_____

_____

_____

PERFORMANCE CHECKLIST 4.7   MEASURING RADIAL-APICAL PULSE

	S	U	COMMENTS
1. Assessed previous pulse rate readings and medical diagnosis.			
2. Determined medications client is taking which may affect pulse rate.			
3. Obtained assistance if possible and washed hands.			
4. Placed the client in position of comfort and explained procedure.			
First Nurse			
5. Cleaned stethoscope properly. Warmed endpiece of stethoscope.			
6. Located apical impulse on chest wall.			
Second Nurse			
7. Located radial pulse using fingertips.			
8. Signaled readiness to first nurse. Each nurse began counting heart rate simultaneously for 1 minute.			
9. Signaled first nurse to stop counting at appropriate time.			
Both Nurses			
10. Compared results.			
11. Washed hands.			
12. Documented results correctly.			

Additional Comments:

_____

_____

_____

_____

_____

Name _____   Specific Skill Performed _____
Date _____   Attempt Number _____
Instructor _____   PASS _____   FAIL _____

PERFORMANCE CHECKLIST 4.8   MEASURING RESPIRATIONS

	S	U	COMMENTS
1. Assessed previous respiratory rate readings and medical diagnosis.			
2. Determined medications client is taking which may affect respirations.			
3. Explained to client that vital signs are being assessed but did not inform client that respirations were being counted.			
4. Observed client's color, and the depth, pattern and rate of respirations. Also checked for other signs of respiratory difficulty.			
5. If respiratory distress is noted, reported findings to appropriate health care professional.			
6. Washed hands.			
7. Documented results correctly.			

Additional Comments:

_____

_____

_____

_____

_____

_____

_____

_____

_____

_____

_____

_____

Name _____   Specific Skill Performed _____
Date _____   Attempt Number _____
Instructor _____   PASS _____   FAIL _____

PERFORMANCE CHECKLIST 4.9   MEASURING BLOOD PRESSURE

	S	U	COMMENTS
1. Assessed previous blood pressure readings and medical diagnosis.			
2. Determined medications client is taking which may affect blood pressure.			
3. Explained procedure to client.			
4. Positioned client's arm correctly and located brachial pulse.			
5. Selected appropriate size cuff and applied cuff correctly 1 to 2 inches above antecubital fossa.			
For a Palpatory Reading			
6. Palpated client's brachial artery as cuff is inflated.			
7. Pumped cuff up 30mmHg higher than point at which client's pulse last felt.			
8. Slowly deflated cuff and identified point at which return of pulse felt.			
For an Auscultatory Reading			
9. Cleaned earpieces and chestpiece of stethoscope.			
10. Applied bell of stethoscope over brachial artery.			
11. Closed valve and inflated cuff to 20 to 30mmHg above point at which pulsation is obliterated.			
12. Deflated cuff by slowly opening valve at rate of 2 to 3mm per second.			
13. Noted point on scale when first beat is heard, "muffling" sound is heard, and last beat is heard.			
14. Completely deflated cuff and removed it from client's arm. Waited 30 to 60 seconds before retaking blood pressure.			

	S	U	COMMENTS
For a Thigh Reading			
15. Placed client in prone position and located the client's popliteal pulse.			
16. Applied appropriate size cuff correctly 1 to 2 inches above bend of knee.			
17. Applied bell of stethoscope directly over popliteal pulse.			
18. Closed valve and inflated cuff 20 to 30mmHg above anticipated systolic reading.			
19. Deflated cuff by slowly opening valve at rate of 2 to 3mmHg per second.			
20. Noted point on scale when first beat is heard and last beat is heard.			
21. Completely deflated cuff and removed from client's leg.			
22. Discussed findings with client, if appropriate, and reported to appropriate personnel.			
23. Washed hands.			
24. Documented results correctly.			

Additional Comments:

_____

_____

_____

_____

_____

_____

_____

_____

_____

_____

Name _____   Specific Skill Performed _____
Date _____   Attempt Number _____
Instructor _____   PASS _____   FAIL _____

PERFORMANCE CHECKLIST 4.10 MEASURING FETAL HEART TONES

	S	U	COMMENTS
1. Assessed previous recordings of fetal heart rate.			
2. Explained procedure to client.			
3. Helped client assume supine position.			
4. Used Leopold maneuvers to locate position of fetus.			
Using a Fetoscope			
5. Cleaned earpieces and abdominal piece of fetoscope and placed fetoscope in your ears.			
6. Placed forehead rest of fetoscope on your forehead. Placed bell of fetoscope firmly on mother's abdomen over area where back of fetus was located.			
7. After locating fetal heart tones, counted fetal heart rate for 1 minute.			
8. Discussed findings with client, if appropriate, and reported to appropriate personnel.			
9. Washed hands.			
10. Documented findings correctly.			
Using a Doppler Ultrasonic Flow Meter			
11. Followed steps 1 through 4 above.			
12. Placed small amount of transmission gel over mother's abdomen where back of fetus was located.			
13. Turned on Doppler ultrasonic flow meter and gently moved it along mother's skin until sound of blood flowing through arteries is heard.			
14. Followed steps 7 through 10 above.			

Name _____   Specific Skill Performed _____

Date _____   Attempt Number _____

Instructor _____   PASS _____   FAIL _____

PERFORMANCE CHECKLIST 4.11 ASSESSING CIRCULATION

		S	U	COMMENTS
1.	Checked results of previous circulation assessments and medical diagnosis.			
2.	Planned to assess portion of extremity distal to point of potential constriction of circulation.			
3.	Assessed for numbness, pain, tingling, or other unusual sensations in distal extremity.			
4.	Assessed color of skin and nailbeds, edema, and movement in distal extremity.			
5.	Correctly assessed capillary refill and temperature of distal extremities.			
6.	Palpated peripheral pulses below area of potential constriction for presence and volume. Graded pulse volume correctly.			
7.	Correctly used Doppler ultrasound flow meter to locate faint or weak pulses. Auscultated sound of blood flowing through arteries.			
8.	If pulses were weak or difficult to find, marked location of pulse with marker.			
9.	Washed hands.			
10.	Notified physician if circulation is poor or deteriorating.			
11.	Documented findings correctly.			

Additional Comments:

_____

_____

_____

_____

_____

_____

_____

PERFORMANCE CHECKLIST 4.12 **ASSESSING NEUROLOGIC STATUS**

	S	U	COMMENTS
1. Noted results of previous neurologic assessments and medical diagnosis.			
2. Explained procedure to client.			
Assessing the Client's Level of Consciousness			
3. Asked questions to assess client's orientation to time, place, and person.			
4. Asked client to squeeze your hand.			
5. Asked client to open eyes. If no response, assessed response to pain.			
Assessing the Client's Pupillary Status			
6. Inspected position and shape of client's pupils.			
7. Darkened room and correctly assessed pupillary reaction to light. Noted direct response as well as consensual response.			
Assessing the Client's Motor Function			
8. Assessed all extremities for movement and strength. If no movement noted, assessed for response to pain.			
9. Correctly tested client's arm strength against gravity.			
10. Washed hands.			
11. Notified physician if assessment indicates deteriorating conditions.			
12. Reassessed neurologic status every 10 to 30 minutes if condition is deteriorating.			
13. Documented results of assessment correctly.			

Additional Comments:

_____

_____

Name _____   Specific Skill Performed _____

Date _____   Attempt Number _____

Instructor _____   PASS _____   FAIL _____

PERFORMANCE CHECKLIST 5.1   MEASURING THE HEIGHT AND WEIGHT OF THE AMBULATORY CLIENT

	S	U	COMMENTS
1. Assessed the client's ability to stand and balance on scale and previous weight.			
2. Asked client to remove shoes. Placed paper towel on scale platform.			
3. Calibrated scale to 0.			
4. Helped client to stand on scale facing balance beam.			
5. Instructed client to remain still and not hold on to scale.			
6. Adjusted weights on scale until beam balances.			
7. Read weight correctly and recorded on notepad.			
8. Helped client turn so that back faces balance beam and instructed client to stand up straight.			
9. Raised and extended height rod over client's head.			
10. Lowered height rod to top of client's head.			
11. Read height correctly and recorded on notepad.			
12. Helped client step down off of scale.			
13. Discussed findings with client.			
14. Washed hands.			
15. Documented client's height and weight correctly.			

Additional Comments:

_____

_____

_____

_____

Name _____   Specific Skill Performed _____
Date _____   Attempt Number _____
Instructor _____   PASS _____   FAIL _____

PERFORMANCE CHECKLIST 5.2   MEASURING THE HEIGHT AND WEIGHT OF THE NONAMBULATORY CLIENT

	S	U	COMMENTS
1. Assessed previous weight and ability to move.			
Bed Scales			
2. Rolled bed scales to edge of bed and locked brakes.			
3. Raised bed to level of scales and locked bed brakes.			
4. Placed sheet on top of scale surface.			
5. Calibrated scale to 0.			
6. Moved client onto scale without injuring client or nurse.			
7. Instructed client to lie still.			
8. Weighed and measured client.			
9. Returned client to bed without injuring client or nurse.			
Hydraulic Lift Bed Scales			
10. Placed lift sheet under client.			
11. Attached hooks or straps of scale to lifter seat and elevated client above bed.			
12. Weighed client.			
13. Slowly lowered client to bed surface and removed lifter seat from under client.			
14. Discussed findings with client if appropriate.			
15. Washed hands.			
16. Documented findings correctly.			

Additional Comments:

_____

_____

Name _____   Specific Skill Performed _____
Date _____   Attempt Number _____
Instructor _____   PASS _____   FAIL _____

PERFORMANCE CHECKLIST 5.3   MEASURING THE WEIGHT OF INFANTS

		S	U	COMMENTS
1.	Assessed infant's previous weight pattern.			
2.	Placed drape on scale.			
3.	Undressed infant and placed infant on scale.			
4.	Held hand over infant's body without touching it while reading infant's weight.			
5.	Discussed findings with parents or caretakers.			
6.	Washed hands.			
7.	Documented weight correctly.			

Additional Comments:

_____

_____

_____

_____

_____

_____

_____

_____

_____

_____

_____

_____

_____

_____

_____

PERFORMANCE CHECKLIST 5.4   MEASURING THE LENGTH OF INFANTS

	S	U	COMMENTS
1. Assessed previous measurements of length.			
2. Placed clean towel on a firm surface.			
3. Laid infant on towel in supine position and kept hand on infant.			
4. Held infant's head at midline and gently extended legs fully.			
5. Stretched tape measure from crown of infant's head to heel of foot.			
6. Read measurement on tape.			
7. Discussed findings with parents or caretakers.			
8. Washed hands.			
9. Documented results correctly.			

Additional Comments:

_____

_____

_____

_____

_____

_____

_____

_____

_____

_____

_____

PERFORMANCE CHECKLIST 5.5   MEASURING HEAD CIRCUMFERENCE

	S	U	COMMENTS
1. Assessed infant's previous head circumference measurements.			
2. Laid infant in supine position on clean towel. Kept hand on infant at all times.			
3. Placed tape measure around fullest part of infant's head over brow.			
4. Read results correctly.			
5. Discussed findings with parents or caretakers.			
6. Washed hands.			
7. Documented results correctly.			

Additional Comments:

_____

_____

_____

_____

_____

_____

_____

_____

_____

_____

_____

_____

_____

_____

Name _____   Specific Skill Performed _____
Date _____   Attempt Number _____
Instructor _____   PASS _____   FAIL _____

PERFORMANCE CHECKLIST 5.6   MEASURING CHEST CIRCUMFERENCE

	S	U	COMMENTS
1. Assessed infant's previous chest circumference measurements.			
2. Laid infant in supine position on clean towel. Kept hand on infant at all times.			
3. Placed tape measure around infant's chest at nipple line.			
4. Read results correctly.			
5. Discussed findings with parents or caretakers.			
6. Washed hands.			
7. Documented results correctly.			

Additional Comments:

_____

_____

_____

_____

_____

_____

_____

_____

_____

_____

_____

_____

_____

Name _____

Date _____

Instructor _____

Specific Skill Performed _____

Attempt Number _____

PASS _____   FAIL _____

PERFORMANCE CHECKLIST 5.7   MEASURING FUNDAL HEIGHT

	S	U	COMMENTS
1. Assessed previous fundal height measurements and weeks of gestation.			
2. Placed client in supine position and draped her to expose the abdomen.			
3. Located symphysis pubis and top of fundus.			
4. Stretched tape measure from symphysis pubis to top of fundus and read results.			
5. Discussed findings with client.			
6. Washed hands.			
7. Documented results correctly.			

Additional Comments:

_____

_____

_____

_____

_____

_____

_____

_____

_____

_____

_____

_____

_____

Name _____   Specific Skill Performed _____
Date _____   Attempt Number _____
Instructor _____   PASS _____   FAIL _____

PERFORMANCE CHECKLIST 5.8   MEASURING ABDOMINAL GIRTH

	S	U	COMMENTS
1. Explained procedure to client.			
2. Placed client in supine or semi-Fowler's position.			
3. Assessed the abdomen for factors which may alter abdominal girth.			
4. Placed tape measure around client's abdomen at largest point and read results.			
5. Marked on client's body where measuring tape lies.			
6. Placed client in position of comfort.			
7. Washed hands.			
8. Documented results correctly.			

Additional Comments:

_____

_____

_____

_____

_____

_____

_____

_____

_____

_____

_____

_____

_____

Name _____

Date _____

Instructor _____

Specific Skill Performed _____

Attempt Number _____

PASS _____   FAIL _____

PERFORMANCE CHECKLIST 5.9   COLLECTING A ROUTINE VOIDED URINE SPECIMEN

	S	U	COMMENTS
1. Assessed client's ability to follow directions and cooperate. Explained procedure to client.			
2. Washed hands and applied gloves.			
3. If female client was menstruating, provided perineal care and inserted tampon.			
4. Instructed client to urinate in clean bedpan or toilet specimen container.			
5. Poured fresh urine into specimen container, put on lid, and labeled correctly. Placed container in biohazard bag and sent immediately to laboratory.			
6. Assessed color and clarity of urine.			
7. Removed gloves and washed hands.			
8. Correctly documented procedure and assessment of urine.			

Additional Comments:

_____

_____

_____

_____

_____

_____

_____

_____

_____

_____

_____

Name _____   Specific Skill Performed _____
Date _____   Attempt Number _____
Instructor _____   PASS _____   FAIL _____

PERFORMANCE CHECKLIST 5.10 COLLECTING A CLEAN-CATCH (MIDSTREAM) URINE SPECIMEN

	S	U	COMMENTS
1. Determined need for test.			
2. Assessed client's ability to follow directions and cooperate. Explained procedure to client.			
3. Provided for client privacy.			
4. Obtained sterile specimen container. Removed lid and placed inside up within easy reach.			
5. Applied sterile gloves. Cleaned urinary meatus correctly with antimicrobial wipes.			
6. If female client was menstruating, placed tampon in vaginal orifice.			
7. Instructed client to void a small amount, stop the stream, and discard urine.			
8. Instructed client to urinate 30 to 50 ml directly into sterile specimen container and finish voiding in toilet.			
9. Placed lid on container without contaminating lid or container.			
10. Assisted client with perineal hygiene.			
11. Removed gloves and washed hands.			
12. Assessed color and clarity of urine.			
13. Labeled specimen correctly, placed in biohazard bag, and sent immediately to laboratory.			
14. Documented procedure and assessment of urine correctly.			

Additional Comments:

_____

_____

_____

_____

Name _____   Specific Skill Performed _____
Date _____   Attempt Number _____
Instructor _____   PASS _____   FAIL _____

PERFORMANCE CHECKLIST 5.11 COLLECTING A URINE SPECIMEN FROM AN INDWELLING CATHETER

	S	U	COMMENTS
1. Determined need for urine specimen.			
2. Explained procedure to client.			
3. Provided for client privacy.			
4. Clamped indwelling catheter tubing just distal to the injection port to allow urine to collect.			
5. Assessed color and clarity of urine in tubing.			
6. Wiped injection port with antimicrobial wipe. Allowed to dry.			
7. Inserted needle into port. Aspirated correct amount of urine into sterile syringe.			
8. Withdrew needle and injected urine into sterile specimen container without contaminating container or urine.			
9. Unclamped catheter tubing and made sure urine is flowing freely.			
10. Placed lid on specimen container and labeled container correctly. Placed specimen in biohazard bag and sent immediately to laboratory.			
11. Washed hands.			
12. Documented procedure and assessment of urine correctly.			

Additional Comments:

_____

_____

_____

_____

_____

_____

_____

Name _____ Specific Skill Performed _____
Date _____ Attempt Number _____
Instructor _____ PASS _____ FAIL _____

PERFORMANCE CHECKLIST 5.12 COLLECTING A URINE SPECIMEN WITH A STRAIGHT CATHETER

	S	U	COMMENTS
1. Checked for physician's order and need for specimen.			
2. Assessed client's ability to follow directions and cooperate. Explained procedure to client.			
3. Provided for patient privacy.			
4. Raised bed to comfortable working height.			
5. Positioned and draped client correctly.			
6. Placed waterproof pad under client's buttocks.			
7. Applied gloves and washed, rinsed, and dried client's genital area.			
8. Removed gloves and washed hands.			
9. Opened sterile catheter insertion kit without contaminating sterile contents.			
10. Removed sterile pad and positioned it appropriately for gender of client.			
11. Placed catheter within sterile field without contaminating it.			
12. Applied sterile gloves correctly.			
13. Placed fenestrated drape over client's genital area.			
14. Poured disinfectant solution over cotton balls.			
15. Lubricated end of catheter appropriately with water-soluble lubricant.			
16. Placed open end of catheter into sterile specimen container.			
17. Cleansed perineal area correctly without allowing recontamination after cleaning.			
18. Picked up disinfectant soaked cotton ball with forceps. Correctly cleansed client's urinary meatus with cotton ball.			
19. Visualized urinary meatus. Gently inserted lubricated end of catheter into meatus without contaminating catheter.			

	S	U	COMMENTS
20. Inserted catheter appropriate distance or until urine began to flow.			
21. Allowed 15 to 20 ml of urine to flow into specimen container and remaining urine to drain into urine receptacle.			
22. Assessed color and clarity of urine.			
23. After bladder is emptied, removed catheter.			
24. Put lid on specimen container, labeled specimen, and placed in biohazard bag. Sent specimen to laboratory immediately.			
25. Washed client's perineal area.			
26. Returned bed to lowest position.			
27. Removed gloves and washed hands.			
28. Disposed of equipment properly.			
29. Documented procedure and assessment of urine correctly.			

Additional Comments:

_____

_____

_____

_____

_____

_____

_____

_____

_____

_____

_____

_____

_____

Name _____ Specific Skill Performed _____

Date _____ Attempt Number _____

Instructor _____ PASS _____   FAIL _____

PERFORMANCE CHECKLIST 5.13 COLLECTING A URINE SPECIMEN FROM A MINICATHETER

	S	U	COMMENTS
1. Checked for physician's order and need for catheterization.			
2. Assessed client's ability to follow directions and cooperate. Explained procedure to client.			
3. Washed hands and provided for client privacy.			
4. Placed bed at comfortable working height or placed client in lithotomy position on exam table. Draped client correctly.			
5. Opened outer wrapper of minicatheter kit without contaminating sterile contents.			
6. Applied sterile gloves.			
7. Opened disinfectant swabs and placed within easy reach.			
8. Pulled 3 to 4 inches of catheter out of test tube and loosened cap on test tube. Placed catheter within easy reach.			
9. Correctly spread labia and cleansed urinary meatus.			
10. Grasped test-tube portion of minicatheter. Inserted tip of catheter into urinary meatus until urine began to flow.			
11. Allowed test tube to fill with urine, then withdrew catheter from urinary meatus.			
12. Pulled catheter out of test tube and discarded appropriately.			
13. Tightened lid on test tube and closed stopper.			
14. Assessed color and clarity of urine.			
15. Returned bed to lowest position. Placed client in position of comfort.			
16. Labeled test tube correctly, placed tube in biohazard bag and sent immediately to laboratory.			
17. Removed gloves and washed hands.			
18. Documented procedure and assessment of urine correctly.			

Name _____   Specific Skill Performed _____
Date _____   Attempt Number _____
Instructor _____   PASS _____   FAIL _____

PERFORMANCE CHECKLIST 5.14 COLLECTING A 24-HOUR URINE SPECIMEN

	S	U	COMMENTS
1. Assessed reason for test and checked physician's order.			
2. Explained procedure to client.			
3. Obtained collection bottle from laboratory.			
4. Posted signs appropriately to remind people that test is in progress.			
5. Instructed client to empty bladder and discarded urine.			
6. Noted beginning time of test.			
7. Instructed client to save all urine for next 24 hours and notify nurse of each voiding.			
8. Kept collection bottle on ice or in refrigerator. Measured urine after each voiding and poured into collection bottle.			
9. Assessed color and clarity of urine after each voiding.			
10. Instructed client to void 15 minutes prior to completion of 24-hour collection period. Poured last voided urine into into collection bottle.			
11. Labeled collection bottle correctly and sent to laboratory.			
12. Documented beginning and ending times of collection and assessment of urine.			

Additional Comments:

_____

_____

_____

_____

_____

_____

_____

Name _____   Specific Skill Performed _____

Date _____   Attempt Number _____

Instructor _____   PASS _____   FAIL _____

PERFORMANCE CHECKLIST 5.15 **COLLECTING A CAPILLARY BLOOD SPECIMEN USING A LANCET OR AN AUTOMATIC PUNCTURE DEVICE**

	S	U	COMMENTS
1. Checked physician's order and explained procedure to client.			
2. Washed hands and applied gloves.			
3. Selected appropriate puncture site and positioned site to facilitate blood flow.			
4. Cleansed site with alcohol swab and allowed to dry.			
5. Punctured site correctly with sterile lancet or automatic puncture device.			
6. Wiped off first two drops of blood with dry gauze or cotton ball.			
7. Collected specimen in appropriate container.			
8. Applied pressure to puncture site with gauze pad or cotton ball.			
9. Applied small adhesive bandage over puncture site.			
10. Properly disposed of lancet.			
11. Checked to make sure bleeding has stopped. Applied pressure to site if necessary.			
12. Removed gloves and washed hands.			
13. Documented procedure correctly.			

Additional Comments:

_____

_____

_____

_____

_____

_____

_____

Name _____   Specific Skill Performed _____
Date _____   Attempt Number _____
Instructor _____   PASS _____   FAIL _____

PERFORMANCE CHECKLIST 5.16 COLLECTING A VENOUS BLOOD SPECIMEN BY VENIPUNCTURE USING A SYRINGE

	S	U	COMMENTS
1. Checked physician's order and explained procedure to client.			
2. Washed hands and applied gloves.			
3. Selected an appropriate puncture site.			
4. Placed site in position to facilitate blood flow.			
5. Asked client to make a fist. Applied tourniquet to extremity above site.			
6. Cleaned site with alcohol swab and allowed to dry.			
7. Anchored vein with thumb of nondominant hand.			
8. Held syringe at $45°$ angle with needle bevel up.			
9. Punctured site and pulled back on plunger to fill syringe with blood.			
10. Immediately loosened tourniquet.			
11. Withdrew syringe and needle. Applied pressure to puncture site.			
12. Applied small adhesive bandage to puncture site.			
13. Carefully transferred blood from syringe to correct collection tube and gently rotated tube. Labeled collection tube correctly.			
14. Properly disposed of syringe and needle.			
15. Placed collection tube in biohazard bag and sent to laboratory.			
16. Removed gloves and washed hands.			
17. Documented procedure correctly.			

Additional Comments:

_____

_____

_____

Name _____   Specific Skill Performed _____
Date _____   Attempt Number _____
Instructor _____   PASS _____   FAIL _____

PERFORMANCE CHECKLIST 5.17 **COLLECTING A VENOUS BLOOD SPECIMEN BY VENIPUNCTURE USING A VACUCONTAINER**

	S	U	COMMENTS
1. Checked physician's order and explained procedure to client.			
2. Washed hands and applied gloves.			
3. Inserted vacucontainer needle into vacucontainer correctly.			
4. Slipped stopper collection tube into vacucontainer without puncturing stopper.			
5. Selected appropriate puncture site and placed site in position to facilitate blood flow.			
6. Asked client to make fist. Applied tourniquet above the selected site.			
7. Cleansed site with alcohol swab and allowed to dry.			
8. Anchored vein with thumb of nondominant hand.			
9. Held vacucontainer with needle at 45° angle and bevel up.			
10. Punctured site and pushed collection tube into puncture stopper.			
11. Immediately loosened tourniquet.			
12. Withdrew vacucontainer needle and applied pressure to site.			
13. Applied small adhesive bandage over puncture site.			
14. Removed and properly disposed of needle.			
15. Removed collection tube from vacucontainer, labeled correctly, and sent to laboratory.			
16. Removed gloves and washed hands.			
17. Documented procedure correctly.			

Additional Comments:

_____

_____

_____

Name _____   Specific Skill Performed _____

Date _____   Attempt Number _____

Instructor _____   PASS _____   FAIL _____

PERFORMANCE CHECKLIST 5.18 COLLECTING A SPUTUM SPECIMEN

	S	U	COMMENTS
1. Assessed client's ability to follow instructions.			
2. Explained procedure and difference between saliva and sputum.			
3. Provided client with appropriate equipment.			
4. Instructed client to rinse mouth with water prior to obtaining specimen.			
5. Instructed client to expectorate sputum into cup without touching inside of cup.			
6. Instructed client to place top on specimen container and call nurse after obtaining specimen.			
7. Applied gloves and took specimen cup from client.			
8. Labeled specimen correctly, placed in biohazard bag, and sent to laboratory.			
9. Observed sputum for color, amount, and consistency.			
10. Removed gloves and washed hands.			
11. Documented procedure and sputum assessment correctly.			

Additional Comments:

_____

_____

_____

_____

_____

_____

_____

_____

PERFORMANCE CHECKLIST 5.19 COLLECTING A STOOL SPECIMEN

	S	U	COMMENTS
1. Assessed for presence of substances which may interfere with test results.			
2. Verified physician's order.			
3. Assessed client's ability to follow instructions and explained procedure to client.			
4. Provided for client privacy.			
5. Instructed client to void prior to collecting specimen. Placed tampon in vaginal orifice if client is menstruating.			
6. Placed client on bedpan or placed clean toilet specimen container in toilet.			
7. Applied gloves and obtained specimen correctly for type of test.			
8. Labeled specimen correctly, put in biohazard bag, and sent to laboratory.			
9. Cleansed client and placed in position of comfort.			
10. Properly cleaned and disposed of equipment.			
11. Removed gloves and washed hands.			
12. Correctly documented procedure and appearance of stool.			

Additional Comments:

_____

_____

_____

_____

_____

_____

_____

_____

Name _____   Specific Skill Performed _____

Date _____   Attempt Number _____

Instructor _____   PASS _____   FAIL _____

PERFORMANCE CHECKLIST 5.20   COLLECTING A URETHRAL SPECIMEN

	S	U	COMMENTS
1. Checked physician's order and reason for test.			
2. Assessed client's ability to follow directions and cooperate. Explained procedure to client.			
3. Positioned and draped client appropriately. Positioned light to increase visualization.			
4. Applied gloves.			
5. Opened culture tube. Held swab with dominant hand.			
6. Clearly visualized urinary meatus to check for drainage.			
7. Inserted swab gently into anterior portion of urethra and obtained drainage at end of swab.			
8. Placed swab in tube with culture medium, squeezed end of tube and pushed swab into medium. Put top on culturette.			
9. Noted color, amount, and odor of drainage.			
10. Washed, rinsed, and dried perineal area.			
11. Removed gloves and washed hands.			
12. Labeled specimen correctly, placed in biohazard bag, and sent to laboratory.			
13. Correctly documented procedure and assessment of drainage.			

Additional Comments:

_____

_____

_____

_____

_____

_____

_____

PERFORMANCE CHECKLIST 5.21 COLLECTING A THROAT SPECIMEN

	S	U	COMMENTS
1. Assessed client's ability to follow directions and cooperate. Explained procedure to client.			
2. Applied gloves.			
3. Instructed client to sit facing you and tilt head back.			
4. Instructed client to open mouth and say "ah".			
5. Illuminated pharyngeal area with penlight. Noted any redness or white exudate.			
6. Held tongue blade in nondominant hand and depressed client's tongue.			
7. With dominant hand, inserted swab and swabbed tonsilar area avoiding oral structures.			
8. Swabbed agar plate or correctly placed swab in culture medium.			
9. Labeled specimen correctly, placed in biohazard bag, and sent to laboratory.			
10. Removed gloves and washed hands.			
11. Documented procedure correctly.			

Additional Comments:

_____

_____

_____

_____

_____

_____

_____

_____

_____

Name _____   Specific Skill Performed _____

Date _____   Attempt Number _____

Instructor _____   PASS _____   FAIL _____

PERFORMANCE CHECKLIST 5.22 COLLECTING A NASAL SPECIMEN

	S	U	COMMENTS
1. Assessed client's ability to follow instructions and cooperate. Explained procedure to client.			
2. Applied gloves.			
3. Instructed client to sit facing you with head tilted back.			
4. Used nasal speculum correctly or pushed tip of nose upward.			
5. Inserted swab through nasal cavity and gently swabbed posterior part of nasal canal.			
6. Placed swab into culture medium tube, squeezed end of tube, pushed swab into medium, and put top on tube.			
7. Labeled specimen correctly, placed in biohazard bag, and sent to laboratory.			
8. Removed gloves and washed hands.			
9. Documented procedure correctly.			

Additional Comments:

_____

_____

_____

_____

_____

_____

_____

_____

_____

PERFORMANCE CHECKLIST 5.23 COLLECTING A WOUND OR LESION CULTURE

	S	U	COMMENTS
1. Determined need for test and explained procedure to client.			
2. Applied gloves.			
3. Positioned area of wound or lesion to facilitate collection of specimen.			
4. Gently swabbed wound or lesion, making sure to swab drainage.			
5. Placed swab correctly in aerobic or anaerobic culture tube.			
6. Labeled specimen correctly, placed in biohazard bag, and sent to laboratory.			
7. Removed gloves and washed hands.			
8. Documented procedure correctly.			

Additional Comments:

_____

_____

_____

_____

_____

_____

_____

_____

_____

_____

_____

Name _____   Specific Skill Performed _____
Date _____   Attempt Number _____
Instructor _____   PASS _____   FAIL _____

PERFORMANCE CHECKLIST 6.1   ASSISTING WITH ABDOMINAL PARACENTESIS

	S	U	COMMENTS
1. Verified physician's order/rationale for procedure.			
2. Verified that informed consent was signed by client.			
3. Discussed procedure with client. Explained/clarified/answered client's questions regarding procedure. Inquired about client allergies (i.e., local anesthetics or antiseptic solutions).			
4. Gathered equipment (paracentesis tray, etc.) and took to bedside.			
Prior to Procedure			
5. Provided privacy for client.			
6. Asked/assisted client to void.			
7. Assessed client condition and gathered pre-procedure data (i.e., B/P, HR, RR, abdominal girth and weight).			
8. Washed hands.			
9. Located equipment for convenient use by physician. Used sterile technique to open and prepare tray.			
10. Assisted client to fully supported upright position in bed or chair.			
11. Placed a B/P cuff on client's arm.			
During Procedure			
12. Assisted physician as needed.			
13. Reassured client during procedure and encouraged him/her to remain in upright position.			
14. Monitored/recorded client's B/P and HR every 15 minutes. Observed client for signs of pallor or sweating.			

	S	U	COMMENTS
After Procedure			
15. Assisted client to comfortable position when procedure completed.			
16. Assessed client's condition and gathered post-procedure data (B/P, HR, RR, abdominal girth and weight).			
17. Labeled fluid specimen and sent to lab according to agency guidelines.			
18. Disposed of equipment according to agency guidelines.			
19. Washed hands.			
20. Monitored client's vital signs, urine output, and dressing according to agency policy/physician's orders (i.e., q 15" x 4, then q 1° x 4).			
21. Documented procedure including assessment data, amount and character of drainage, client tolerance and disposition of specimen. Reported client condition to appropriate persons.			

Additional Comments:

_____

_____

_____

_____

_____

_____

_____

_____

_____

_____

_____

Name _____

Date _____

Instructor _____

Specific Skill Performed _____

Attempt Number _____

PASS _____   FAIL _____

PERFORMANCE CHECKLIST 6.2   **ASSISTING WITH BONE MARROW ASPIRATION AND BIOPSY**

	S	U	COMMENTS
1. Checked physician's order/rationale for the procedure.			
2. Verified that consent form was signed by client.			
3. Gathered equipment (bone marrow tray, etc.) for later use.			
4. Discussed procedure with client. Explained what to expect before and after the procedure.			
5. Inquired about client bleeding disorders and allergies (i.e., local anesthetics or antiseptic solutions).			
6. Checked client's medications for any that may interfere with clotting.			
7. Assessed client condition and gathered pre-procedure data (i.e., VS).			
8. Administered pre-operative medication if ordered.			
9. Took equipment to bedside (if not already done).			

Prior to Procedure

	S	U	COMMENTS
10. Provided privacy and positioned client appropriately for access to aspiration site (supine for sternum and anterior crest or prone for posterior crest).			
11. Washed hands.			
12. Located equipment for convenient use by physician. Used sterile technique to open and prepare tray.			

During Procedure

	S	U	COMMENTS
13. Reassured client throughout procedure and assisted physician as needed.			

	S	U	COMMENTS
After Procedure			
14. When procedure completed, labeled specimens carefully and sent them to laboratory.			

15. Post-procedure site care:
   a. for aspiration, applied direct pressure for 5 to 15 minutes followed by small dressing.
   b. for biopsy, applied direct pressure as above but followed by a pressure dressing for 60 minutes.			

16. Assisted client to recumbent position with pressure on the site.			
17. Assessed client's condition and gathered post-procedure data (VS, bleeding at puncture site, etc.).			
18. Reiterated post-procedure expectations.			
19. Disposed of equipment according to agency policy.			
20. Washed hands.			
21. Documented procedure including assessment data, client education, client tolerance of procedure and disposition of specimen(s). Reported client's condition to appropriate persons.			

Additional Comments:

_____

_____

_____

_____

_____

_____

_____

_____

_____

_____

PERFORMANCE CHECKLIST 6.3   **ASSISTING WITH BRONCHOSCOPY**

	S	U	COMMENTS
1. Checked physician's order/rationale for the procedure and verified that consent form was signed by client.			
2. Gathered appropriate equipment if procedure to be done at bedside.			
3. Discussed procedure with client. Explained what to expect before and after the procedure.			
4. Inquired about client allergies (i.e., local anesthetic spray).			
5. Ensured that client had nothing by mouth (NPO) since midnight.			
6. Had client void. Collected pre-operative assessment data (i.e., vital signs, etc.). Had client remove dentures, contact lenses, and/or prosthesis.			
7. Administered pre-op medication as ordered and prepared client for transport to exam site (if not at bedside).			
Prior to Procedure			
8. Provided privacy and positioned client appropriately (supine, lateral or semi-Fowler's) with neck hyperextended.			
9. Washed hands and placed equipment for convenient use by the physician.			
During Procedure			
10. Monitored client's vital signs during the procedure.			
11. Reassured client throughout procedure and assisted physician as needed.			
12. When procedure completed, sent specimen(s) to lab and disposed of equipment according to agency policy.			
13. Washed hands.			

	S	U	COMMENTS
After Procedure			
14. Checked client's gag reflex after procedure and at intervals (according to agency policy) until gag reflex returned.			
15. Kept client NPO until gag reflex returned.			
16. After cough and gag reflex returned, administered ice chips/ fluids by mouth.			
17. Observed client post-operatively for signs of adverse responses.			
18. Documented procedure including assessment data, client education, client response to the procedure, and disposition of specimen(s). Reported client condition to appropriate persons.			

Additional Comments:

_____

_____

_____

_____

_____

_____

_____

_____

_____

_____

_____

_____

_____

_____

_____

Name _____   Specific Skill Performed _____
Date _____   Attempt Number _____
Instructor _____   PASS _____   FAIL _____

PERFORMANCE CHECKLIST 6.4   **ASSISTING WITH AN ELECTROCARDIOGRAM**

	S	U	COMMENTS
1. Checked physician's order/rationale for the procedure.			
2. Gathered equipment and took to the bedside.			
3. Discussed procedure with client. Explained to client what to expect (i.e., 10 to 15 minutes, painless).			
Prior to Procedure			
4. Gathered assessment data as appropriate (i.e., age, sex, height, weight, B/P, pulse, symptoms, medications, deformities, etc.).			
5. Provided privacy and assisted client to supine position.			
During Procedure			
6. Placed electrodes (limb and chest) appropriately and attached the lead wires.			
7. Requested client to remain still during procedure.			
8. Recorded electrocardiogram as ordered (i.e., 12-lead) and according to manufacturer's operational guidelines.			
After Procedure			
9. When procedure completed, removed leads/paste and assisted client to comfortable position.			
10. Washed hands and removed equipment.			
11. Placed ECG on chart (or as appropriate according to agency policy).			
12. Documented the procedure, including assessment data and client tolerance. Reported client's condition to appropriate persons.			

Additional Comments:

_____

_____

Name _____   Specific Skill Performed _____

Date _____   Attempt Number _____

Instructor _____   PASS _____   FAIL _____

PERFORMANCE CHECKLIST 6.5   ASSISTING WITH ENDOSCOPY

	S	U	COMMENTS
1. Checked physician's order/rationale for the procedure.			
2. Verified that consent form was signed by client.			
3. Gathered equipment/supplies if procedure to be done on unit. If done off unit, checked schedule to confirm time, etc.			
4. Discussed procedure with client. Explained what to expect before and after procedure.			
5. Inquired about client allergies (i.e., medications, etc.).			
6. Verified that pre-op requirements were carried out (i.e., NPO, bowel prep, assessment data, pre-op med, etc.).			
7. Ensured that client was appropriately dressed for the procedure (hospital gown, no underwear). Transported client to procedure site if appropriate.			
Prior to Procedure			
8. Took/recorded client's vital signs.			
9. Started intravenous infusion if ordered.			
10. Provided privacy and assisted client to appropriate position for procedure.			
During Procedure			
11. Monitored client's vital signs per protocol and as needed.			
12. Reassured client throughout procedure.			
13. Assisted physician as needed.			
After Procedure			
14. Assisted client back to bed and into a position of comfort and safety.			

	S	U	COMMENTS
15. Assessed client status (level of consciousness, vital signs, adverse reactions) according to agency policy/physician's orders (i.e., q 15" x 4, then q 1° x 4).			
16. Notified physician of changes in client's baseline status from pre-operative status.			
17. Documented procedure including assessment data, analgesia given, client's reaction and disposition of specimens. Reported client's condition to appropriate persons.			

Additional Comments:

_____

_____

_____

_____

_____

_____

_____

_____

_____

_____

_____

_____

_____

_____

_____

_____

_____

_____

Name _____   Specific Skill Performed _____
Date _____   Attempt Number _____
Instructor _____   PASS _____   FAIL _____

PERFORMANCE CHECKLIST 6.6   **ASSISTING WITH A LIVER BIOPSY**

	S	U	COMMENTS
1. Checked physician's order/rationale for the procedure.			
2. Checked medication record for meds that interfere with clotting.			
3. Verified that consent form was signed by client.			
4. Discussed procedure with client. Explained what to expect before and after procedure, including activity restrictions. Inquired about allergies and bleeding disorders.			
5. Verified that pre-op requirements were carried out (i.e., NPO, pre-op meds, etc.).			
6. Gathered equipment and took to bedside.			
Prior to Procedure			
7. Took client's vital signs.			
8. Provided privacy and assisted client to appropriate position (supine with right arm behind head and over left shoulder) with abdomen exposed.			
9. Washed hands.			
10. Placed equipment for convenient use by physician. Used sterile technique to open tray.			
11. Put on clean gloves (for self-protection) before procedure.			
12. Informed client of physician's activity and requested client's cooperation (i.e., lie still, hold breath during needle insertion, etc.).			
13. Reassured client during procedure and assisted physician as needed.			
After Procedure			
14. Applied pressure to puncture site immediately following the procedure (per agency guidelines or as ordered).			
15. Applied sterile dressing to puncture site.			

	S	U	COMMENTS
16. Assisted client to right lateral position with pillow/towel under puncture site. Instructed client to remain there for 3 hours.			
17. Labeled/sent specimens to lab according to agency policy.			
18. Disposed of equipment according to agency policy.			
19. Washed hands.			
20. Assessed client condition (VS, dressing) q 10 to 20 minutes (until stable for 2 hours with no evident bleeding).			
21. Documented procedure including assessment data, meds given, client's reaction and disposition of specimen. Reported client condition to appropriate persons.			

Additional Comments:

_____

_____

_____

_____

_____

_____

_____

_____

_____

_____

_____

_____

_____

_____

_____

_____

PERFORMANCE CHECKLIST 6.7   ASSISTING WITH A LUMBAR PUNCTURE

	S	U	COMMENTS
1. Checked physician's order/rationale for the procedure.			
2. Verified that consent form was signed by client.			
3. Discussed procedure with client. Explained what to expect before and after procedure. Inquired about allergies (i.e., local anesthetics/antiseptics).			
4. Gathered equipment (including extra pillows) and took to bedside/exam site.			
Prior to Procedure			
5. Had client empty urinary bladder.			
6. Provided privacy and assisted client to bed or exam table if appropriate.			
7. Washed hands.			
8. Placed equipment for convenient use by physician. Used sterile technique to open tray. Added additional supplies to sterile field if needed.			
9. Assisted client to edge of bed/table and to assume appropriate position (i.e., lateral recumbent, back bowed, knees flexed to abdomen, head bent with chin on chest). Placed a pillow between client's legs and another under head.			
During Procedure			
10. Informed client of physician's activity. Instructed client to take slow deep breaths during needle insertion.			
11. Reassured client during procedure and assisted physician as needed (i.e., Queckenstedt's test).			
12. Carefully labeled the specimens sequentially.			

	S	U	COMMENTS
After the Procedure			
13. Assisted client to appropriate position (i.e., prone for 2 hours). Advised client of subsequent position changes (per agency protocol or as ordered).			
14. Assessed puncture site and applied adhesive bandage.			
15. Encouraged client to drink plenty of fluids.			
16. Labeled and sent CSF specimen to laboratory according to agency policy.			
17. Disposed of equipment according to agency policy.			
18. Washed hands.			
19. Documented procedure, including assessment data, and character of CSF, client's reaction and disposition of the specimen. Reported client condition to appropriate persons.			

Additional Comments:

_____

_____

_____

_____

_____

_____

_____

_____

_____

_____

_____

_____

_____

Name _____   Specific Skill Performed _____
Date _____   Attempt Number _____
Instructor _____   PASS _____   FAIL _____

PERFORMANCE CHECKLIST 6.8   **ASSISTING WITH PROCTOSIGMOIDOSCOPY**

	S	U	COMMENTS
1. Checked physician's order/rationale for the procedure.			
2. Verified that consent form was signed by client.			
3. Discussed procedure with client. Explained what to expect before and after procedure.			
4. Verified that pre-op requirements were carried out (i.e., enema/suppository, pre-op meds, hospital gown without underwear, vital signs, etc.).			
5. Gathered equipment and took to bedside if appropriate (or transported client to exam area at appropriate time).			
Prior to Procedure			
6. Provided privacy and assisted client to appropriate position on bed or exam table (i.e., knee-chest, left lateral with anus exposed).			
7. Washed hands.			
8. Placed equipment for convenient use by physician. Opened proctoscopy tray and other needed supplies.			
9. Put on exam gloves.			
During Procedure			
10. Informed client of physician's activity and offered reassurance.			
11. Assisted physician as needed.			
12. Assessed client for changes in status during procedure (i.e., pallor, diaphoresis, vital signs, etc.).			
After the Procedure			
13. Wiped client's anus with gauze to remove lubricant and fecal material.			
14. Assisted client to position of comfort.			

	S	U	COMMENTS
15. Labeled/sent specimens to lab per agency policy.			
16. Disposed of equipment according to agency guidelines.			
17. Assessed client condition (VS, pain, drainage) per protocol or as ordered (i.e., q 15 minutes x 4, then 1 hour x 4).			
18. Documented procedure including assessment data, meds given, client's reaction and disposition of specimen. Reported client's condition to appropriate persons.			

Additional Comments:

_____

_____

_____

_____

_____

_____

_____

_____

_____

_____

_____

_____

_____

_____

_____

_____

_____

_____

Name _____   Specific Skill Performed _____

Date _____   Attempt Number _____

Instructor _____   PASS _____   FAIL _____

PERFORMANCE CHECKLIST 6.9   **ASSISTING WITH THORACENTESIS**

	S	U	COMMENTS
1. Checked physician's order/rationale for the procedure.			
2. Verified that consent form was signed by client.			
3. Discussed procedure with client. Explained what to expect before and after the procedure. Inquired about client allergies (i.e., local anesthetics, antiseptic).			
4. Verified that pre-procedure requirements were carried out (i.e., chest x-ray, ultrasound, client assessment, VS, etc.).			
5. Gathered equipment and took to bedside.			
Prior to Procedure			
6. Provided privacy and assisted client to appropriate position (sitting on side of bed, straddling a chair, lying on unaffected side with head of bed elevated with chest exposed).			
7. Washed hands.			
8. Placed equipment for convenient use by physician. Used sterile technique to open thoracentesis tray and added supplies if needed.			
9. Ensured that lighting was adequate for performance of the procedure.			
During Procedure			
10. Informed client of physician's activity, requested client cooperation (i.e., be very still, don't cough, etc.) and offered reassurance.			
11. Assessed client for changes in status during procedure (i.e., respiratory distress, increased heart rate, signs of hypoxia, etc.).			
After the Procedure			
12. Applied pressure to needle insertion site and applied sterile dressing.			

	S	U	COMMENTS
13. Assisted client to position of comfort.			
14. Checked with physician regarding post-procedure chest x-ray of client.			
15. Labeled/sent specimens to lab per agency policy.			
16. Disposed of equipment according to agency guidelines.			
17. Washed hands.			
18. Assessed client's condition as needed for signs of adverse responses (i.e., respiratory distress, chest discomfort, cough, blood-tinged sputum, faintness, vertigo, rapid pulse, cyanosis, etc.).			
19. Documented procedure including assessment data, meds given, x-rays performed, client's reaction, and disposition of specimens. Reported client's condition to appropriate persons.			

Additional Comments:

_____

_____

_____

_____

_____

_____

_____

_____

_____

_____

_____

_____

_____

Name _____   Specific Skill Performed _____
Date _____   Attempt Number _____
Instructor _____   PASS _____   FAIL _____

PERFORMANCE CHECKLIST 6.10   MEASURING BLOOD GLUCOSE

	S	U	COMMENTS
1. Checked client's chart for history of diabetes and/or indication for need for finger stick blood glucose determination.			
2. Gathered equipment (i.e., reagent strips, instrument to read blood sugar, lancet, etc.) and took to bedside.			
3. Discussed procedure with client. Explained what to expect before and after procedure.			
4. Put on clean exam gloves.			
5. Used appropriate technique to obtain a blood specimen from client's finger (i.e., lancet, safety lancet, etc.).			
6. Checked expiration date on reagent strip bottle before removing one strip. Observed strip for discoloration.			
7. Touched one large drop of blood to completely cover reagent test pad(s) without smearing the blood.			
8. Covered puncture site with dry gauze and applied pressure (or had client apply pressure).			
9. Followed manufacturer's directions regarding developing time and handling of blood drop/test pad (i.e., wipe, don't wipe, rinse off, etc.).			
10. **For Visual Reading**: Under a good light source, compared the test pad colors to color scale on test strip bottle.			
11. **For Instrument Reading**: Followed directions in operation manual for blood glucose meter to obtain reading from test strip.			
12. Disposed of soiled equipment per protocol.			
13. Removed gloves and washed hands.			
14. Explained results to client if appropriate.			
15. Recorded results on client's chart and reported results to appropriate person if indicated.			

Name _____

Date _____

Instructor _____

Specific Skill Performed _____

Attempt Number _____

PASS _____   FAIL _____

PERFORMANCE CHECKLIST 6.11   **PERFORMING AN AUDIOMETRIC EXAMINATION**

	S	U	COMMENTS
1. Gathered equipment (i.e., audiometer, etc.) and selected a quiet room in which to perform examination.			
2. Placed audiometer on table and arranged chairs (examiner, examinee) appropriately.			
3. Ensured that audiometer was functioning.			
4. Seated client facing away from the audiometer and instructed client to give a signal when a sound is heard (i.e., raise hand at onset, lower it when stops). Varied instructions according to client capabilities.			
5. Placed earphones on client's head and ensured proper fit.			
6. Administered test tone (i.e., 1,000 Hz, 40 dB) in each ear and observed client.			
7. Turned intensity to 25 dB and tested each of the client's ears at the following frequencies: 1,000 Hz, 2,000 Hz, 4,000 Hz, 8,000 Hz, and 500 Hz. Completed test on one ear before moving to other ear.			
8. Observed/recorded client response after each frequency. Kept a record of missed frequencies.			
9. If hearing not satisfactory, examined client's ear with otoscope (i.e., checked for presence of excessive cerumen, otitis media, etc.).			
10. Explained results to client or sent letter home to child's parents with test results and recommendations. Documented findings in client's chart.			
11. Made appropriate referrals based on findings. Scheduled client for re-screening before referral to hearing specialist if appropriate.			

Additional Comments:

_____

_____

_____

Name _____   Specific Skill Performed _____
Date _____   Attempt Number _____
Instructor _____   PASS _____   FAIL _____

PERFORMANCE CHECKLIST 6.12   MEASURING HEMATOCRIT (CAPILLARY METHOD)

	S	U	COMMENTS
1. Checked client's chart/history to learn previous HCT reading and to determine rationale for test (i.e., conditions that alter HCT, etc.).			
2. Explained procedure to client.			
3. Gathered supplies, washed hands, and put on clean exam gloves.			
4. Used appropriate technique to collect a blood sample from a finger or heel stick (i.e., lancet, safety lancet, etc.) and followed instructions for filling capillary tube.			
5. Filled two capillary tubes three-quarters full. Covered puncture site with gauze/tissue and had client apply pressure if necessary.			
6. Sealed one end of each capillary tube with sealing clay.			
7. Placed capillary tube into slot in HSM centrifuge head (sealed end toward periphery) and the other tube opposite it.			
8. Secured head cover. Closed and latched HSM centrifuge cover.			
9. Set timer on centrifuge (at least 5 minutes at 1,000 to 1,300 revolutions per minute) and started machine. Followed manufacturer's operational instructions.			
10. At end of spin cycle, waited until spontaneous rotation of centrifuge head ceased before lifting the outside cover and unfastening the head cover.			
11. Removed the capillary tubes and noted appearance of the plasma. Used a spirocrit (hematocrit reader) to read percent volume of packed red cells. Followed manufacturer's instructions if precalibrated capillary tubes were used.			
12. Disposed of equipment according to agency policy.			
13. Removed gloves and washed hands.			
14. Discussed findings with client if appropriate.			
15. Documented results in client record.			

Name _____   Specific Skill Performed _____
Date _____   Attempt Number _____
Instructor _____   PASS _____   FAIL _____

PERFORMANCE CHECKLIST 6.13   TESTING STOOL FOR OCCULT BLOOD

	S	U	COMMENTS
1. Checked client's diet/chart for foods/meds taken in last 48 to 72 hours that may affect outcome of test.			
2. Helped client implement dietary or medication changes if appropriate (i.e., in preparation for test).			
3. Gathered equipment and took to bedside.			
4. Discussed test with client (i.e., specimen collection, etc.) and requested client cooperation.			
5. Provided privacy for client and assisted client to bedpan, bedside commode, or bathroom as appropriate for specimen collection.			
6. Put on gloves.			
7. Collected stool specimen appropriately.			
8. Followed instructions on guiac test kit to prepare stool for test. Used different area of specimen to obtain second stool smear.			
9. Closed front flap, turned kit over and opened flap on reverse side to expose test areas.			
10. Followed instructions to apply guiac developer to test box and control site (i.e., 2 gtts. test box, 1 gtt. to control area).			
11. Waited appropriate length of time (i.e., 60 seconds) to compare test to control.			
12. Discarded soiled supplies according to agency policy.			
13. Cleansed client if needed and assisted him/her to position of comfort.			
14. Removed gloves and washed hands.			
15. Explained results of test to client if appropriate.			
16. Documented results of test in client's record/chart.			

Additional Comments:

_____

_____

Name _____
Date _____
Instructor _____   PASS _____   FAIL _____

PERFORMANCE CHECKLIST 6.14   SCREENING FOR LICE

		S	U	COMMENTS
1.	Determined need for inspection for lice (i.e., exposure to others, etc.).			
2.	Provided privacy for client.			
3.	Put on clean examination gloves.			
4.	Separated hair shafts and inspected client's scalp, and appropriate skin surfaces for presence of lice, nits (eggs) and evidence of bites and pustules.			
5.	Did not allow self to become contaminated during inspection (i.e., stood away from client to prevent contact with lice).			
6.	Disposed of gloves according to agency policy (i.e., airtight container to be burned, etc.).			
7.	Washed hands.			
8.	Explained results to client or sent letter home to child's parents/caretaker.			
9.	Made recommendation/referral regarding treatment.			
10.	Scheduled a follow-up appointment for re-check after treatment (or scheduled re-check if client in-house).			

Additional Comments:

_____

_____

_____

_____

_____

_____

_____

_____

_____

PERFORMANCE CHECKLIST 6.15   TESTING URINE

	S	U	COMMENTS
1. Checked client's chart for medical diagnosis (past and present) of conditions that may cause altered test results.			
2. Provided client with container for routine voided urine specimen. Assisted client as needed.			
3. Obtained bottle of urine dipsticks and checked expiration dates. Removed a strip, checked for discoloration and re-capped bottle.			
4. Put on clean examination gloves before handling specimen.			
5. Observed urine for color, clarity, sediment, odor, and other characteristics.			
For Visual Reading of Results			
6. Completely immersed dipstick reagent pads in fresh urine.			
7. Tapped edge of dipstick against rim of specimen container to remove excess urine and removed it immediately.			
8. While holding the strip in a horizontal position, compared the test areas to the corresponding color chart on the bottle label at the specified time.			
9. Discarded the soiled equipment/specimen according to agency policy.			
10. Removed gloves and washed hands.			
11. Explained results to client if appropriate.			
12. Documented test results on client's chart including urine characteristics.			
For Instrument Reading of Results			
13. Used urine chemistry analyzer recommended by dipstick manufacturer and followed directions in operations manual.			

Name _____   Specific Skill Performed _____
Date _____   Attempt Number _____
Instructor _____   PASS _____   FAIL _____

PERFORMANCE CHECKLIST 6.16   SCREENING FOR PHENYLKETONURIA

	S	U	COMMENTS
1. Determined age of child and types of PKU test (blood or urine) to be done.			
2. Discussed test with client's family if appropriate.			
3. Gathered equipment and prepared for use.			
4. Put on clean gloves.			
5. Used appropriate technique to collect a blood specimen from child's heel.			
6. Saturated designated areas on PKU test paper with blood from heel stick.			
7. Labeled the specimen and sent it to the laboratory.			
8. Discarded soiled equipment according to agency policy.			
9. Removed gloves and washed hands.			
10. Counseled client's family regarding results and referral to physician for further examination if appropriate.			
11. Documented procedure on client's record including information provided to family.			

Additional Comments:

_____

_____

_____

_____

_____

_____

_____

_____

_____

PERFORMANCE CHECKLIST 6.17   **SCREENING FOR SICKLE HEMOGLOBIN**

	S	U	COMMENTS
1. Determined need for test (i.e., history of sickle cell disease in family).			
2. Discussed test with client's family.			
3. Gathered equipment and prepared for use.			
4. Put on examination gloves.			
5. Used appropriate technique to collect a blood specimen from finger.			
6. Soaked a large area on sickle cell test paper with blood (i.e., area the size of a quarter).			
7. Labeled the specimen and sent to laboratory.			
8. Discarded soiled equipment according to agency policy.			
9. Removed gloves and washed hands.			
10. Counseled client's family regarding results and referral to physician for further examination if appropriate.			
11. Documented procedure on client's record including information provided to family.			

Additional Comments:

_____

_____

_____

_____

_____

_____

_____

_____

Name _____   Specific Skill Performed _____
Date _____   Attempt Number _____
Instructor _____   PASS _____   FAIL _____

PERFORMANCE CHECKLIST 6.18   **MEASURING THE SPECIFIC GRAVITY OF URINE**

	S	U	COMMENTS
1. Assessed client chart/history for conditions (past and present) that may cause altered urinary specific gravity (i.e., renal disease, DM, DI, diuretics, etc.).			
2. Assessed client's hydration status (i.e., skin turgor, I & O, mucous membranes, etc.).			
3. Discussed procedure with client. Provided specimen container and instructed client in self-collection of 20 ml. uncontaminated urine.			
4. Provided for privacy and assisted client as needed.			
5. Obtained equipment and prepared for use.			
6. Put on clean exam gloves and checked accuracy of the urinometer (i.e., checked specific gravity of water).			
7. Filled cylinder two-thirds full with urine.			
8. Placed urinometer in cylinder and waited for movement to stop.			
9. At eye level, determined highest point of urine contact on scale.			
10. Discarded the urine and cleaned the cylinder and urinometer.			
11. Removed gloves and washed hands.			
12. Documented procedure results in client's record.			

Additional Comments:

_____

_____

_____

_____

_____

_____

_____

_____

Name _____   Specific Skill Performed _____

Date _____   Attempt Number _____

Instructor _____   PASS _____   FAIL _____

PERFORMANCE CHECKLIST 6.19   PERFORMING TUBERCULIN SKIN TESTS

	S	U	COMMENTS
1. Asked client if he/she tests positive to TB skin test or had BCG vaccination in past. Asked about recent viral illness.			
2. Explained test to client.			
3. Obtained appropriate TB skin test and prepared for use.			
4. Put on clean gloves. Selected/cleaned test site.			
For Tine Test			
5. Opened the tine test and pressed the prongs firmly on client's forearm.			
For Mantoux Test			
6. Administered 0.1 ml. of PPD into dermis of client's arm using appropriate technique for giving intradermal injections.			
After Administration of TB Skin Test			
7. Discarded soiled equipment according to agency policy.			
8. Removed gloves and washed hands.			
9. Noted location of TB skin test on client's arm (i.e., circled area with marking pen) and instructed client regarding test site evaluation in 48 to 72 hours. Instructed client to return if appropriate.			
10. After 48 to 72 hours, measured induration present at site of puncture mark. Explained the results to client.			
11. Made appropriate referral for further testing/treatment if test was positive.			
12. Recorded the procedure, including assessment data, test results and referrals on client's record.			

Name _____   Specific Skill Performed _____
Date _____   Attempt Number _____
Instructor _____   PASS _____   FAIL _____

PERFORMANCE CHECKLIST 6.20   **SCREENING VISION**

	S	U	COMMENTS
1. Determined need for vision testing (i.e., mass screening, clinic, etc.).			
2. Gathered equipment necessary for vision screening.			
3. Selected well-lighted area with at least 20 feet of distance from the wall.			
4. Hung Snellen chart(s) on wall with referral line at client's eye level. Removed or covered any other distractions on wall.			
5. Placed tape on floor 20 feet from vision charts.			
6. Explained test to client and discussed purpose for test.			
7. If client had corrective lenses, asked him/her to wear them during test.			
8. Covered/had client cover right eye (i.e., index card, cupped hand, etc.) but instructed client to keep both eyes open during test.			
9. Held pointer vertically below symbol(s) in first line that client could see clearly and had client read line.			
10. Had client read progressively smaller lines on the eye chart until they could no longer read a majority of the symbols in the line (i.e., no more than 2 errors per line).			
11. Observed client behavior for squinting, tearing of eyes, tilting of head or leaning forward.			
12. Determined client's visual acuity (from chart).			
13. Repeated actions for left side.			
14. If client read 20/20 line and did not wear glasses, requested that they read the line with the +2 diopter lens on.			
15. Scheduled a re-screen if client's vision not satisfactory.			
16. Referred client to appropriate eye specialist if vision not satisfactory on second screening.			
17. Documented the results of the vision screen(s) and referrals on client's record.			

Name _____   Specific Skill Performed _____
Date _____   Attempt Number _____
Instructor _____   PASS _____   FAIL _____

PERFORMANCE CHECKLIST 6.21   ASSISTING WITH A VAGINAL EXAMINATION

	S	U	COMMENTS
1. Determined need for procedure (i.e., checked client's chart/record, physician's orders, etc.).			
2. Explained procedure to client. Inquired about previous Pap smears and medical management.			
3. Asked client to empty her bladder, undress, and put on gown.			
4. Assisted client to supine position on exam table.			
5. Placed drape over client and adjusted stirrups.			
6. Assisted client to lithotomy position with feet positioned in stirrups. Ensured that client was properly draped with perineum exposed.			
7. Directed light source toward client's perineum.			
8. Placed waste receptacle near the foot of the examining table.			
9. Arranged necessary equipment on Mayo stand and placed it for convenient use (i.e., between assistant and examiner).			
10. Put on gloves and provided gloves for examiner.			
11. Handed examiner a vaginal speculum moistened with warm water.			
For a Pap Smear			
12. Handed examiner a wooden spatula and a cotton-tipped applicator for collection of cervical scraping, endocervical sample and vaginal smear.			
13. Held slide (on frosted end) to allow examiner to smear the vaginal specimen on the slide.			
14. Sprayed the slide lightly with cytology fixative.			
15. Labeled specimen and set aside for later processing.			

	S	U	COMMENTS
For a Wet Prep			
16. Handed a cotton-tipped applicator to examiner for collection of client's vaginal secretions.			
17. Placed 2 to 3 drops of saline in a test tube.			
18. Placed cotton-tipped applicator with the specimen into the saline solution.			
19. Labeled the specimen and sent to laboratory for immediate examination.			
For a Gonorrhea Culture			
20. Handed examiner a cotton-tipped applicator for collection of specimen from client's endocervical canal.			
21. If agar plate used, streaked agar with specimen-laden applicator, covered plate and sealed in airtight bag with a carbon dioxide tablet. If culture bottle used, held capped bottle in upright position. Opened bottle just prior to use and used appropriate technique to inoculate the medium in a timely manner.			
22. Discarded swab according to agency policy.			
23. Labeled specimen and sent to lab for incubation.			
24. Placed soiled speculum in disinfectant solution to soak.			
For a Bimanual Examination			
25. Placed a small amount of water-soluble lubricant on examiner's fingers for the bimanual examination.			
26. Instructed client to breathe deeply and relax her pelvic muscles as examination is performed.			
After Examination			
27. Disposed of soiled equipment according to agency policy.			
28. Assisted client to get off examination table.			
29. Provided client with towelette for personal hygiene.			

	S	U	COMMENTS
30. Washed hands.			
31. Documented procedure in client's record including client reaction and disposition of specimen.			

Additional Comments:

_____

_____

_____

_____

_____

_____

_____

_____

_____

_____

_____

_____

_____

_____

_____

_____

_____

_____

Name _____   Specific Skill Performed _____
Date _____   Attempt Number _____
Instructor _____   PASS _____   FAIL _____

PERFORMANCE CHECKLIST 7.1   **HELPING THE CLIENT TO MOVE UP IN BED**

	S	U	COMMENTS
1. Reviewed activity orders and contraindications to moving client.			
2. Assessed client's self-care abilities and ability to follow directions.			
3. Explained procedure to client.			
4. Locked wheels on bed, lowered side rails.			
5. Lowered head of bed and adjusted bed to comfortable working height.			
6. Removed pillows placing one against the head of the bed.			
7. Positioned tubes to prevent accidental removal or kinking.			
8. Stood facing head of bed diagonally in a stance to provide a wide base of support and prevent back injury.			
9. Placed one hand under client's shoulders and one under client's hips.			
10. Asked client to flex knees, place feet flat on the mattress and assist you on the count of three. Correctly used trapeze or draw sheet if available.			
11. Shifted your weight forward as you helped the client move.			
12. Helped client to assume good body alignment.			
13. Assessed tubes for proper functioning.			
14. Replaced call light and placed bed in a position of safety.			
15. Discarded soiled laundry. Washed hands.			
16. Documented procedure correctly.			

Additional Comments:

_____

_____

_____

_____

Name _____   Specific Skill Performed _____

Date _____   Attempt Number _____

Instructor _____   PASS _____   FAIL _____

PERFORMANCE CHECKLIST 7.2   HELPING THE CLIENT TO SIT ON THE SIDE OF THE BED

	S	U	COMMENTS
1. Assessed physician's order and client's medical diagnosis.			
2. Assessed client's ability to sit up.			
3. Locked bed wheels. Adjusted bed to comfortable working height.			
4. Lowered side rails and moved client to side of bed.			
5. Raised head of bed.			
6. Faced opposite side of bed.			
7. Placed one hand under client's shoulders and one under client's hips.			
8. Pivoted client to sitting position while shifting your weight.			
9. Supported client until stable.			
10. Lowered bed to lowest position. Placed footstool under client's feet.			
11. When ready, helped client to lie down by reversing procedure.			
12. Helped client to assume position of good alignment and repositioned tubing.			
13. Washed hands.			
14. Documented procedure and response of client.			

Additional Comments:

_____

_____

_____

_____

_____

_____

_____

Name _____   Specific Skill Performed _____
Date _____   Attempt Number _____
Instructor _____   PASS _____   FAIL _____

PERFORMANCE CHECKLIST 7.3   **TRANSFERRING THE CLIENT FROM A BED TO A STRETCHER**

	S	U	COMMENTS
1. Reviewed diagnosis and activity orders. Assessed mobility level, limitations, level of consciousness, placement of tubes, and ability to follow directions.			
2. Gathered appropriate equipment.			
3. Explained procedure to client. Fan-folded linen to foot of bed.			
4. Locked wheels on bed. Raised bed to level of stretcher.			
Assisting the Client Who Is Mobile			
5. Positioned the stretcher next to the bed. Locked wheels on stretcher.			
6. Lowered head of bed and loosened top sheet.			
7. Stood on side of stretcher opposite bed.			
8. Asked client to move to the edge of the bed and then to the center of the stretcher using correct body mechanics.			
Assisting the Client Who Is Immobile, Confused, Sedated, or Unresponsive			
9. Obtained the help of three additional nurses who should stand on the side of the bed to which the client is to be moved.			
10. Placed client's arms across the abdomen. Loosened drawsheet and rolled it toward client.			
11. Each nurse supported a part of the client's body and grasped a part of the drawsheet.			
12. On the count of three, nurses lifted and moved the client to the side of the bed closest to the stretcher.			
13. Positioned stretcher next to bed and locked wheels.			
14. With two nurses positioned on side of stretcher opposite bed and one on opposite side of bed, grasped the drawsheet.			
15. On count of three, nurses lifted and moved client to stretcher.			

	S	U	COMMENTS
After Transfer of Both the Mobile and Immobile Client			
16. Helped client to assume good body alignment and repositioned tubing.			
17. Raised side rails on stretcher.			
18. Washed hands.			
19. Documented procedure correctly.			

Additional Comments:

_____

_____

_____

_____

_____

_____

_____

_____

_____

_____

_____

_____

_____

_____

_____

_____

_____

Name _____   Specific Skill Performed _____
Date _____   Attempt Number _____
Instructor _____   PASS _____   FAIL _____

PERFORMANCE CHECKLIST 7.4   **TRANSFERRING THE CLIENT FROM A BED TO A CHAIR OR WHEELCHAIR**

	S	U	COMMENTS
1. Reviewed diagnosis and activity orders. Assessed level of consciousness, placement of tubes, and ability to follow directions.			
2. Explained procedure to client.			
3. Locked bed wheels and placed bed in lowest position. Positioned chair at correct angle to bed.			
4. Positioned tubes on same side of bed as chair and ensured slack in tubing.			
5. Helped client to sitting position on side of the bed nearest chair.			
6. Assumed forward-backward stance facing client. Slid client's buttocks to edge of bed.			
7. Grasped center of ambulation belt or supported client correctly and securely.			
8. Asked client to stand while shifting your weight from forward to backward.			
9. Encouraged client to stand up straight with your knees against client's forward weaker knee.			
10. Assessed for presence of orthostatic hypotension and, if present, returned to bed.			
11. Asked client to place near hand on far arm of chair and pivot on the balls of the feet.			
12. Asked client to step back until legs touch chair seat and grasp chair's other arm with other hand.			
13. Lowered client into chair. Repositioned and reconnected any tubing.			
14. Assessed client for comfort and proper positioning.			
15. Washed hands.			
16. Reversed procedure for returning client to bed.			
17. Documented client's change in position and tolerance of activity.			

Name _____   Specific Skill Performed _____
Date _____   Attempt Number _____
Instructor _____   PASS _____   FAIL _____

PERFORMANCE CHECKLIST 7.5   **TRANSFERRING THE CLIENT WITH A HYDRAULIC LIFT**

	S	U	COMMENTS
1. Reviewed diagnosis and activity orders. Assessed mobility level, limitations, level of consciousness, tubes, and ability to follow directions.			
2. Checked weight capacity of the lift.			
3. Explained procedure to client. Applied ambulation belt if needed.			
4. Locked wheels of the bed and positioned chair close to bed.			
5. Positioned tubes on side of bed where chair is placed. Ensured slack in tubing.			
6. Rolled client on side and positioned sling of lift correctly under client.			
7. Made sure sling is centered and folded client's arms on chest.			
8. Lowered side rail and positioned lift on side of bed with chair.			
9. Carefully lifted frame and passed it over client while positioning lift base under bed.			
10. Lowered frame around client and secured sling to hooks on frame. Covered client with sheet or blanket.			
11. Raised lift by cranking handle on frame. Secured client with safety belt.			
12. Wheeled client to destination and positioned lift over chair.			
13. Lowered client into chair and disconnected sling from lift.			
14. Repositioned and reconnected tubing if necessary.			
15. Placed client in position of comfort and safety and assessed for tolerance of move.			
16. Washed hands.			
17. Documented procedure and client's tolerance.			

PERFORMANCE CHECKLIST 7.6   **LOGROLLING THE CLIENT**

	S	U	COMMENTS
1. Assessed client's medical diagnosis and need for logrolling.			
2. Explained procedure to client.			
3. Raised bed to comfortable working height and locked wheels.			
4. Obtained assistance and placed nurse on each side of the bed.			
5. Used drawsheet to slide client to edge of bed.			
6. Placed pillow lengthwise between client's legs.			
7. Positioned client's arms correctly and raised bed rails.			
8. Nurses moved to side of bed toward which the client will turn.			
9. Nurses worked in coordinated manner to roll client in one motion to side-lying position.			
10. Placed client in correct body alignment and placed wedge against client's back.			
11. Flexed client's top leg at knee and placed pillow between knee and lower leg.			
12. Washed hands.			
13. Documented procedure correctly.			

Additional Comments:

_____

_____

_____

_____

_____

_____

_____

_____

Name _____   Specific Skill Performed _____

Date _____   Attempt Number _____

Instructor _____   PASS _____   FAIL _____

PERFORMANCE CHECKLIST 7.7   **MOVING THE CLIENT TO THE SUPINE POSITION**

	S	U	COMMENTS
1. Assessed client's medical diagnosis and need for supine position.			
2. Asked client to lie on back in middle of bed.			
3. Aligned client's body with straight spine in center of bed and client's head toward top of bed.			
4. Placed trochanter roll on either side of client's hips and thighs.			
5. Placed pillow under client's head, neck, and upper shoulders.			
6. Elevated client's hands and arms correctly on pillows.			
7. Placed pillows under client's lower legs.			
8. If desired, positioned client with knees slightly bent to relieve pressure on lower back. Avoided pressure directly on popliteal area.			
9. Placed soles of feet firmly against footboard with toes pointing straight up.			
10. Assessed client frequently for correct body alignment and areas of pressure on skin. Alternated position as needed.			
11. Washed hands.			
12. Documented procedure correctly.			

Additional Comments:

_____

_____

_____

_____

_____

_____

_____

_____

Name _____   Specific Skill Performed _____

Date _____   Attempt Number _____

Instructor _____   PASS _____   FAIL _____

PERFORMANCE CHECKLIST 7.8   **MOVING THE CLIENT TO THE PRONE POSITION**

	S	U	COMMENTS
1. Assessed client's medical diagnosis and ability to lay in prone position.			
2. Assessed for tubes or attachments and made plans for type and method of move.			
3. Obtained necessary assistance and equipment.			
4. Explained procedure to client and provided for privacy.			
5. Adjusted bed to comfortable working height, locked wheels and lowered side rails.			
6. Placed lift sheet under client and changed soiled linen if necessary.			
7. Placed client flat in supine position. Removed all pillows and positioning devices.			
8. Moved client to side of bed opposite direction of planned turn.			
9. Placed pillows on bed next to client to protect proper pressure points.			
10. Adjusted client's gown so that it is not wrinkled or constricting at neckline.			
11. Placed client's arms flat against body with palms next to thighs.			
12. Stood on side of bed toward which client will turn. Supported client's head and legs.			
13. Rolled client over arm into face-down position in coordinated fashion.			
14. Assessed client's respiratory status. Turned head to side and placed small pillow under face.			
15. Positioned arms flexed at elbows with palms down.			
16. Adjusted waist and leg pillows as needed.			
17. Placed small pillows or rolls between axilla and clavicle.			
18. Checked that client's feet are hanging over the end of the mattress or are supported with ankles at 90° angle.			

	S	U	COMMENTS
19. Assessed for proper body alignment.			
20. Covered client, raised side rails.			
21. Placed call light within reach and assessed client's comfort.			
22. Periodically changed client's arm positions. Encouraged coughing and deep breathing.			
23. Washed hands.			
24. Documented procedure correctly.			

Additional Comments:

_____

_____

_____

_____

_____

_____

_____

_____

_____

_____

_____

_____

_____

_____

_____

_____

Name _____   Specific Skill Performed _____
Date _____   Attempt Number _____
Instructor _____   PASS _____   FAIL _____

PERFORMANCE CHECKLIST 7.9   **MOVING THE CLIENT TO THE SIDE-LYING POSITION**

	S	U	COMMENTS
1. Reviewed client's medical diagnosis and any contraindications to positioning.			
2. Began with client in supine position. Removed all pillows and positioning devices.			
3. Moved client to side of bed opposite one client will face when turned.			
4. Placed small pillow at waist on side to which client will turn.			
5. Placed client's head pillow so it will support head and neck after turn.			
6. Moved to opposite side of bed and positioned client's shoulder and elbow nearest you correctly.			
7. Placed client's other arm and hand across abdomen. Placed far leg across near leg.			
8. Placed your fingers around client's body at shoulder and hip or used drawsheet and rolled client toward you.			
9. Positioned client's lower shoulder by gently pulling it slightly toward you.			
10. Adjusted waist and head pillows as necessary. Elevated upper arm and hand on pillow.			
11. Placed pillow under upper leg and foot for support and correct degree of flexion.			
12. Used sandbag to hold client's lower foot in place with ankle at 90°.			
13. Covered client. Assessed comfort and correct body alignment.			
14. Washed hands.			
15. Documented procedure correctly.			

Additional Comments:

_____

_____

Name _____

Date _____

Instructor _____

Specific Skill Performed _____

Attempt Number _____

PASS _____   FAIL _____

PERFORMANCE CHECKLIST 7.10 **MOVING THE CLIENT TO THE SIMS POSITION**

	S	U	COMMENTS
1. Reviewed the client's medical diagnosis and contraindications to moving.			
2. Assessed tubes or attachments and made plans for type and method of move.			
3. Assessed need for assistance. Obtained necessary equipment.			
4. Explained procedure to client and provided for privacy.			
5. Positioned client on back and removed all pillows, positioning devices, and linen.			
6. Moved client to right side of bed.			
7. Correctly placed pillows in line with the client's body to allow for support.			
8. Placed both arms flat against body with palms next to thighs. Placed right leg over left leg.			
9. Cupped hands around client's shoulder and hip. Rolled client toward you, over the arm, and halfway between side-lying and prone in a coordinated motion.			
10. Checked client's nose and mouth to be certain airway is open and client is breathing. Placed small pillow or pad under one side of face.			
11. Checked that spine is parallel with side of bed and shoulders are in line with hips.			
12. Retracted and hyperextended lower shoulder and placed arm in position of comfort behind client's body.			
13. Checked that right arm is comfortably flexed with arm and torso supported on pillows.			
14. Checked that hips and legs are in proper alignment with right leg supported on pillows.			
15. Placed sole of left foot firmly against sandbag to maintain angle at 90°.			

	S	U	COMMENTS
16. Covered client as needed, placed call light in reach, and raised side rails.			
17. Washed hands.			
18. Documented procedure correctly.			

Additional Comments:

_____

_____

_____

_____

_____

_____

_____

_____

_____

_____

_____

_____

_____

_____

_____

_____

_____

_____

_____

_____

_____

Name _____

Date _____

Instructor _____

Specific Skill Performed _____

Attempt Number _____

PASS _____   FAIL _____

PERFORMANCE CHECKLIST 7.11   **MOVING THE CLIENT TO THE TRENDELENBURG POSITION**

	S	U	COMMENTS
1. Reviewed client's medical diagnosis and contraindications to moving.			
2. Positioned client on back.			
3. Elevated the lower portion of the bed 45° while maintaining the client's spine and bed frame in a straight line.			
4. Placed a small pillow between the client's head and the head board.			
5. Covered the client, placed call light in reach, and raised the side rails.			
6. Washed hands.			
7. Documented procedure correctly.			

Additional Comments:

_____

_____

_____

_____

_____

_____

_____

_____

_____

_____

_____

_____

Name _____   Specific Skill Performed _____
Date _____   Attempt Number _____
Instructor _____   PASS _____   FAIL _____

PERFORMANCE CHECKLIST 7.12   MOVING THE CLIENT TO THE REVERSE TRENDELENBURG POSITION

	S	U	COMMENTS
1. Reviewed the client's medical diagnosis and contraindications to moving.			
2. Positioned client on back.			
3. Raised upper portion of the bed 30° and lowered the foot of the bed while maintaining the client's spine and bed's frame in a straight line.			
4. Placed a footboard at the end of the bed and positioned client's feet against it.			
5. Placed a small pillow under the client's head.			
6. Covered the client, placed the call light in reach, and raised the side rails.			
7. Washed hands.			
8. Documented the procedure correctly.			

Additional Comments:

_____

_____

_____

_____

_____

_____

_____

_____

_____

_____

_____

Name _____   Specific Skill Performed _____
Date _____   Attempt Number _____
Instructor _____   PASS _____   FAIL _____

PERFORMANCE CHECKLIST 7.13   MOVING THE CLIENT TO THE FOWLER POSITION

	S	U	COMMENTS
1. Reviewed the client's medical diagnosis and contraindications to moving.			
2. Positioned client on back.			
3. Pulled client up in bed using proper body mechanics.			
4. Used the bed control to raise the head of the bed to the proper angle.			
5. Placed a small pillow behind the client's head and under each arm with client's fingers extended.			
6. Used a footboard to keep client's ankles flexed at 90°.			
7. Covered client, placed call light in reach, and raised side rails.			
8. Washed hands.			
9. Documented procedure correctly.			

Additional Comments:

_____

_____

_____

_____

_____

_____

_____

_____

_____

_____

_____

Name _____   Specific Skill Performed _____
Date _____   Attempt Number _____
Instructor _____   PASS _____   FAIL _____

PERFORMANCE CHECKLIST 7.14   **ASSISTING THE CLIENT WITH AMBULATION**

	S	U	COMMENTS
1. Reviewed the client's medical diagnosis and contraindications to moving.			
2. Cleared the path of obstacles and locked the wheels of the bed.			
3. Explained the procedure to the client.			
4. Lowered the bed to the lowest position.			
5. Helped the client to sit on the side of the bed and to put on slippers and housecoat.			
6. Applied ambulation belt if needed and helped client to stand.			
7. Supported client under axilla and around waist. Walked slightly behind and to the side of the client.			
8. After walk is completed, helped the client back to bed.			
9. Positioned the client for comfort and safety.			
10. Washed hands.			
11. Documented the procedure and the client's tolerance.			

Additional Comments:

_____

_____

_____

_____

_____

_____

_____

_____

_____

Name _____   Specific Skill Performed _____

Date _____   Attempt Number _____

Instructor _____   PASS _____   FAIL _____

PERFORMANCE CHECKLIST 7.15   ASSISTING THE CLIENT WITH THE USE OF A CANE

	S	U	COMMENTS
1. Assessed the client's knowledge and readiness to learn.			
2. Instructed the client to use the cane on the unaffected side close to the body and to inspect the rubber tip daily for worn places.			
3. Helped the client put on shoes and stand to measure correct cane height.			
4. Explained and demonstrated correct cane-walking gait.			
5. Helped the client to practice and answered any questions correctly.			
6. Assessed client's ability to use cane.			
7. Helped the client return to bed and positioned for comfort and safety.			
8. Washed hands.			
9. Documented procedure correctly.			

Additional Comments:

_____

_____

_____

_____

_____

_____

_____

_____

_____

_____

Name _____   Specific Skill Performed _____
Date _____   Attempt Number _____
Instructor _____   PASS _____   FAIL _____

PERFORMANCE CHECKLIST 7.16   ASSISTING THE CLIENT WITH THE USE OF CRUTCHES

	S	U	COMMENTS
1. Assessed the client's knowledge and readiness to learn.			
2. Assisted client in putting on shoes and standing.			
3. Measured crutches for correct length.			
4. Instructed client to bear the body weight on the hands and inspect the rubber tips daily for worn places.			
5. Instructed client on different gait patterns and assisted in choosing one.			
6. Instructed client on the correct technique for going up and down stairs, sitting and standing.			
7. Demonstrated selected gait and techniques for using crutches.			
8. Helped the client practice.			
9. Assessed client's ability to use crutches and the selected gait.			
10. Helped the client return to bed and positioned for comfort and safety.			
11. Washed hands.			
12. Documented the procedure correctly.			

Additional Comments:

_____

_____

_____

_____

_____

_____

_____

_____

Name _____
Date _____
Instructor _____

Specific Skill Performed _____
Attempt Number _____
PASS _____   FAIL _____

PERFORMANCE CHECKLIST 7.17   ASSISTING THE CLIENT WITH THE USE OF A WALKER

	S	U	COMMENTS
1. Assessed the client's knowledge and readiness to learn.			
2. Helped the client to put on shoes and stand to measure for correct length.			
3. Instructed the client on picking up the walker and moving it forward, walking to the walker one step at a time.			
4. Instructed the client to inspect the rubber tips daily for worn places.			
5. Demonstrated the correct walking technique.			
6. Helped the client to practice.			
7. Assessed the client's ability to use the walker.			
8. Helped the client return to bed and placed in a position of comfort and safety.			
9. Washed hands.			
10. Documented the procedure correctly.			

Additional Comments:

_____

_____

_____

_____

_____

_____

_____

_____

_____

Name _____

Date _____

Instructor _____

Specific Skill Performed _____

Attempt Number _____

PASS _____   FAIL _____

PERFORMANCE CHECKLIST 8.1   **ASSISTING WITH RANGE-OF-MOTION EXERCISES**

	S	U	COMMENTS
1. Checked client's chart and assessed client for contraindications to the procedure.			
2. Raised client's bed to comfortable working level and lowered side rail. Discussed procedure with client and explained what to expect.			
3. Assisted client to supine position and removed pillow from under client's head. Covered client with bath blanket and fan-folded bed covers to foot of bed.			
Supine Position Exercises			
4. Performed ROM exercises of client's neck.			
5. Performed shoulder ROM exercises.			
6. Performed elbow ROM exercises.			
7. Performed ROM exercises of client's wrists and elbows.			
8. Performed ROM exercises of the fingers and thumb.			
9. Performed ROM exercises of client's hip and knee.			
10. Performed ROM exercises of client's ankle and foot.			
11. Performed ROM exercises of the toes.			
Prone Position Exercises			
12. Positioned client in prone position. Performed ROM exercises of the neck.			
13. Performed ROM exercises of the shoulder.			
14. Performed ROM exercises of the hip.			
15. Performed ROM exercises of the knee.			
16. Assisted client to Fowler's position and performed ROM exercises of the trunk.			

	S	U	COMMENTS
After the ROM Exercises			
17. Assisted client to position of comfort, raised the side rails, and lowered the bed to low position.			
18. Assessed the client's comfort and physical condition.			
19. Documented the procedure including assessment data and client's reaction.			

Additional Comments:

_____

_____

_____

_____

_____

_____

_____

_____

_____

_____

_____

_____

_____

_____

_____

_____

_____

_____

Name _____   Specific Skill Performed _____

Date _____   Attempt Number _____

Instructor _____   PASS _____   FAIL _____

PERFORMANCE CHECKLIST 8.2   **ASSISTING WITH ANTIEMBOLI HOSE**

	S	U	COMMENTS
1. Checked chart for physician's order/rationale for/type of antiemboli hose to be applied.			
2. Explained procedure/purpose to client and what to expect after application.			
3. Assisted client to supine position and measured client's leg appropriately for the type of hose ordered.			
4. Obtained correct size hose and took to bedside (with powder).			
5. Assisted client to supine position and exposed legs. Generously applied powder (or cornstarch) to client's legs and feet.			
6. Opened package and made sure that stockings were "inside out." Placed hand inside one stocking (deep enough to grasp toe of stocking).			
7. Used other hand (palm down on instep) to grasp the toes of one of the client's feet.			
8. With first hand (inside inverted hose), grasped the toes distally and began placement of the stocking. Put inverted stocking over toes (and hand holding toes). Then removed hands from inside the stocking.			
9. Held both sides of stocking and pulled the inverted stocking over the toes.			
10. Gently but firmly pulled the stocking from toes to heel (in one motion).			
11. Held onto each side of stocking and pulled it past the client's ankle.			
12. Continued to pull stocking up client's leg (in 2-inch increments) until entire stocking placed.			
13. Repeated steps 6-12 for other leg.			
14. Ensured that stockings were smooth and wrinkle-free.			
15. Washed hands.			
16. Documented the procedure.			

	S	U	COMMENTS
After Application of Antiemboli Hose			
17. Checked client's legs frequently to ascertain proper fit (i.e., circulation, swelling, rolling of hose, etc.)			
18. Removed both stockings for 30 minutes twice a day. Assessed/ bathed/dried/powdered legs and reapplied stockings.			
19. Washed and dried the stockings as needed.			

Additional Comments:

_____

_____

_____

_____

_____

_____

_____

_____

_____

_____

_____

_____

_____

_____

_____

Name _____   Specific Skill Performed _____

Date _____   Attempt Number _____

Instructor _____   PASS _____   FAIL _____

PERFORMANCE CHECKLIST 8.3   **ASSISTING WITH POSTOPERATIVE LEG EXERCISES**

	S	U	COMMENTS
1. Assessed client/obtained baseline data (i.e., condition(s) that may contraindicate leg exercises, muscle strength and mobility, knowledge regarding postoperative exercises).			
2. Explained/clarified and taught exercises to client before operation. Had client perform a return demonstration.			
After Operation			
3. Assessed client prior to beginning post-op exercises (i.e., vital signs, Homan's sign, post-op condition, comfort level).			
4. Medicated client prior to exercises if appropriate.			
5. Assisted client to supine position. Raised bed to comfortable working height if passive exercises anticipated.			
6. Asked client to perform feet exercises (5 to 7 times): a. rotation of each ankle b. inversion and eversion of each ankle c. alternate dorsiflexion and plantar flexion of each foot			
7. Asked client to perform leg exercises (5 to 7 times): a. slowly bend leg until heel is close to buttocks b. straighten leg until knee is flat on bed c. repeat with opposite leg			
8. Reminded/instructed client that exercises should be performed every two hours during waking hours.			
9. Assessed client's condition following exercises (i.e., vital signs, activity tolerance, mobility and muscle strength).			
10. Positioned client for comfort and ensured that bed was in low position and side rails up (if appropriate).			
11. Documented exercises and assessment data.			

Additional Comments:

_____

_____

_____

Name _____   Specific Skill Performed _____
Date _____   Attempt Number _____
Instructor _____   PASS _____   FAIL _____

PERFORMANCE CHECKLIST 8.4   **SPECIAL MATTRESSES, BEDS, AND POSITIONING DEVICES**

	S	U	COMMENTS
Pressure-relieving Devices			
1. Egg Crate/Foam Mattress a. placed foam mattress on top of client's mattress and covered with a single sheet.			
2. Sheepskin a. placed sheepskin directly against client's skin (under buttocks, around heels or elbows, etc.).			
3. Flotation Pads a. placed flotation pad under client's bony prominences (i.e., as cushion in chair, wheel chair, etc.).			

4. Alternating Pressure Air Mattress
   a. placed air mattress over client's mattress and covered with a single sheet.
   b. followed manufacturer's instruction to initiate/maintain alternating pressure in mattress.			

5. Special Beds a. followed manufacturer's instruction to initiate/maintain operation of special bed.			
Positioning Devices			

6. Pillows, Bolsters, and Trochanter Rolls
   a. placed pillows and/or bolsters appropriately to maintain client in good body alignment.
   b. obtained/made and placed trochanter rolls appropriately to prevent external rotation of client's hips.			

7. Hip Abduction Wedge a. appropriately placed hip abduction wedge between client's legs to maintain hips in abducted position.			
8. Bed Cradles a. placed/anchored appropriate bed cradle to client's bed to lift to sheets off client's skin.			

	S	U	COMMENTS

9. Hand Rolls
   a. obtained/made and placed hand rolls in client's palms.
   b. checked to see that client's fingers were in correct
      anatomic alignment around hand roll.			

10. Footboards
   a. placed/anchored footboard at foot of client's bed.
   b. ensured that client's feet rested firmly against footboard
      before replacing top covers over footboard.			

11. Sandbags
   a. obtained/placed sandbags appropriately to maintain client's
      body parts in good body alignment.			

Documentation			
12. Appropriately documented in client's record the use/placement of assist devices including any relevant assessment data.			

Additional Comments:

_____

_____

_____

_____

_____

_____

_____

_____

_____

_____

_____

_____

_____

_____

Name _____

Date _____

Instructor _____

PERFORMANCE CHECKLIST 8.5   USING A STRYKER WEDGE TURNING FRAME

	S	U	COMMENTS
1. Before turning, assessed client (i.e., skin, neurologic status, level of knowledge and anxiety regarding turn, tolerance for new position).			
Preparing to Turn the Client			
2. Solicited help.			
3. Provided needed/appropriate nursing care before turning.			
4. Placed all lines/tubes (i.e., IV, N/G) at head of bed. Used extension tubing if needed. Place urinary collection bag on mattress beside client.			
5. Locked the wheels of the frame.			
Turning the Client From a Supine to a Prone Position			
6. Removed top linen. Placed pillow lengthwise over client's legs.			
7. Placed client's arms at his/her sides. Removed arm boards out of way.			
8. Placed small pillow/folded towel beside client's head to prevent head movement during turn.			
9. Put clean linen on anterior frame.			
10. Placed anterior frame over client and tightened knurled nut (at head of frame).			
11. Closed/locked turning ring over anterior frame.			
12. Fastened the foot and tightened the nuts on the anterior turning ring.			
13. Secured the restraining straps.			
14. Removed the lock pin (at head of frame).			
15. Pulled out the red turning lock knob (on turning ring).			

	S	U	COMMENTS
16. Stood on narrow edge of wedge, grasped turning handle and informed client before beginning turn.			
17. Smoothly turned frame toward client's right.			
18. Pushed in silver lock knob (on turning ring).			
19. Removed the restraining straps and posterior frame.			
20. Replaced the lock pin (at head of frame).			
21. Replaced arm boards and repositioned lines (i.e., IV, N/G) and collection devices appropriately.			
22. Ensured that client was properly positioned (i.e., good body alignment), then placed a restraining strap around him/her.			
23. Covered client with sheet and/or blanket as needed.			
Turning the Client From the Prone to the Supine Position			
24. Followed steps 1 through 5 when preparing to turn client.			
25. Removed covers and positioned necessary incontinence pads and sheepskin over client's buttocks. Placed small pillow in client's lumbar curve.			
26. Place clean linen on posterior frame.			
27. Positioned posterior frame over client and secured it appropriately.			
28. Followed steps 11 through 23 to complete the turn to the supine position.			
Following the Turning Process			
29. After turning, assessed the client's neurologic status.			
30. Documented the procedure in the client's record including pre/post assessment data and client response to turning.			

Additional Comments:

_____

_____

_____

_____

Name _____   Specific Skill Performed _____
Date _____   Attempt Number _____
Instructor _____   PASS _____   FAIL _____

PERFORMANCE CHECKLIST 8.6   **CAST CARE**

	S	U	COMMENTS
1. Checked chart for type of injury and type of cast.			
2. Put on clean gloves if appropriate (i.e., drainage present) before handling cast.			
3. Elevated client's extremity appropriately to assist venous return.			
4. Encouraged drying of cast (i.e., open to air, repositioned client frequently, etc.).			
5. Assessed client's circulation and neurovascular status in affected area appropriately (i.e., q 30 min. x 4 hrs., then q 1 hr. x 24 hrs., then q 4 hrs.).			
6. Periodically checked edges of cast for roughness. When cast dry, padded the edges as needed.			
7. Checked for evidence of bleeding (including underneath cast) and marked area appropriately.			
8. Assessed for swelling.			
9. Assessed for pressure area under cast.			
10. Assessed for odors and signs/symptoms of infection.			
11. Assessed circulation distal to cast.			
12. Assessed for signs/symptoms of compartment syndrome. Notified physician immediately if signs/symptoms present.			
13. Instructed client to refrain from inserting anything into cast.			
14. Assisted client with pain management.			
15. Performed ROM exercises for client (unless contraindicated).			
16. Used appropriate methods to keep cast clean.			
17. Washed hands following cast care.			
18. Documented cast care as appropriate including assessment data and performance of ROM exercises.			

Name _____   Specific Skill Performed _____
Date _____   Attempt Number _____
Instructor _____   PASS _____   FAIL _____

PERFORMANCE CHECKLIST 8.7   **CARING FOR THE CLIENT IN TRACTION**

	S	U	COMMENTS
1. Obtained baseline assessment data (i.e., neurovascular status, vital signs, comfort level, nutritional status, skin condition, etc.).			
2. Determined type of traction being used.			
3. Determined type of position client is allowed to assume.			
For all Traction			
4. Assessed neurovascular status of areas distal to injury as ordered/ according to agency policy and as needed.			
5. Ensured that client was in good body alignment in middle of the bed with traction lines correctly placed.			
6. Did not allow client's feet to touch end of bed.			
7. Ensured that all ropes remained in pulleys and that weights were hanging free.			
8. Did not remove weights without physician's orders. When removed/ reapplied, ensured that they were lowered smoothly and slowly.			
9. Evaluated affected and dependent skin areas every 3 to 4 hours.			
10. Provided skin protection devices as needed (i.e., heel and elbow protectors, sheepskin, etc.) and kept linen wrinkle-free.			
11. Provided/encouraged client to use overhead trapeze to assist with movement in bed.			
12. Assisted client with passive/active ROM exercises as appropriate. Assisted with isometric/isotonic exercise as ordered.			
13. Provided a fracture pan for client's elimination needs and monitored frequency or ease of client's bowel movements.			
14. Made bed from head to foot and did not tuck in top linen.			
15. Provided for adequate hydration, nutrition, and respiratory hygiene every shift.			

	S	U	COMMENTS
For Skin Traction			
16. Provided appropriate care to client's skin under the covered traction areas and to dependent areas.			
17. Assessed mobility of joints affected by traction if appropriate.			
18. Maintained appropriate pressure with wraps and splints.			
For Skeletal Traction			
19. Assessed pin insertion site for: a. signs/symptoms of infection b. loosening			
20. Uses aseptic technique to provide care to insertion site as ordered.			
Documentation			
21. Recorded assessment data/observations and care provided in client's record.			

Additional Comments:

_____

_____

_____

_____

_____

_____

_____

_____

_____

_____

_____

_____

Name _____ Specific Skill Performed _____
Date _____ Attempt Number _____
Instructor _____ PASS _____ FAIL _____

PERFORMANCE CHECKLIST 9.1 **APPLYING RESTRAINTS**

	S	U	COMMENTS
1. Assessed need for restraints and type of restraint needed.			
2. Obtained physician's order if necessary.			
3. Obtained necessary equipment and assistance if needed.			
4. Washed hands.			
5. Explained purpose of restraints to client and family.			
6. Inspected skin and neurovascular status of limb before applying restraint.			
7. Padded bony prominences.			
8. Correctly applied restraint and fastened to appropriate part of bed frame.			
9. Checked that client is in good anatomical body alignment.			
10. Ensured that client can be released quickly in an emergency.			
11. Took precautions to prevent complications from restraints such as decreased circulation, decreased muscle movement, and skin breakdown.			
12. Documented the procedure correctly.			

Additional Comments:

_____

_____

_____

_____

_____

_____

_____

_____

Name _____   Specific Skill Performed _____
Date _____   Attempt Number _____
Instructor _____   PASS _____   FAIL _____

PERFORMANCE CHECKLIST 10.1   ASSISTING WITH ORAL HYGIENE

	S	U	COMMENTS
1. Assessed client's self-care abilities and explained procedure to client.			
2. Positioned client in an upright position or, if unresponsive, positioned on side with the bed at a comfortable working height.			
3. Washed hands and applied gloves.			
4. Placed waterproof pads over bed linens and garments.			
5. Filled drinking cup with water. Allowed client to rinse mouth with water and expectorate into emesis basin.			
6. Observed for respiratory difficulties.			
7. Placed small amount of toothpaste on toothbrush.			
8. Held toothbrush at a 45° angle while moving in circular, vibrating motion.			
9. Brushed all exposed areas as well as inner and outer surfaces of all teeth correctly.			
10. Gently brushed client's tongue avoiding stimulation of gag reflex.			
11. Allowed client to expectorate and rinse mouth as needed. Assisted in wiping client's mouth.			
12. Flossed client's teeth correctly.			
13. Allowed client to rinse mouth with water and/or mouthwash.			
14. Used protective ointment on lips if necessary.			
15. Emptied emesis basin, cleaned toothbrush under running water.			
16. Placed client in position of comfort and lowered bed to safe height.			
17. Removed gloves and washed hands.			
18. Documented procedure correctly.			

Name _____   Specific Skill Performed _____
Date _____   Attempt Number _____
Instructor _____   PASS _____   FAIL _____

PERFORMANCE CHECKLIST 10.2   **ASSISTING WITH DENTURE CARE**

	S	U	COMMENTS
1. Assessed self-care abilities of client.			
2. Explained procedure to client.			
3. Gathered appropriate equipment.			
4. Washed hands and applied gloves.			
5. Asked client to remove dentures or removed them gently from the client's mouth.			
6. Assessed dentures for worn linings, plaque, food debris, and broken or cracked areas.			
7. Placed dentures in denture cup filled with water or denture cleaning solution.			
8. Placed paper towel or washcloth in the bottom of the sink with a small amount of water.			
9. Placed small amount of toothpaste or denture paste on toothbrush.			
10. Holding each denture over sink, grasped each denture, one at a time, in palm of one hand while brushing with the other hand.			
11. Rinsed each denture and placed in clean denture cup.			
12. Allowed client to rinse mouth with warm water and mouthwash.			
13. Cleaned oral mucosa and tongue with soft nylon brush or toothettes.			
14. Massaged client's gums with gloved thumb and index finger.			
15. Replaced dentures in client's mouth and checked to be certain dentures resealed, or placed in a clean, clearly labeled denture cup with fresh water.			
16. Removed and disposed of gloves. Washed hands.			
17. Documented procedure correctly.			

Name _____

Date _____

Instructor _____

Specific Skill Performed _____

Attempt Number _____

PASS _____   FAIL _____

PERFORMANCE CHECKLIST 10.3   PROVIDING EYE CARE FOR THE CLIENT WHO DOES NOT BLINK

	S	U	COMMENTS
1. Assessed client's eye for abnormalities.			
2. Reviewed chart for information regarding eye care and condition.			
3. Placed towel under client's head.			
4. Turned client's head to one side.			
5. Washed hands and applied gloves.			
6. Used wet, warm washcloth without soap to clean client's eye from inner canthus to outer canthus.			
7. If eye was crusted, left warm, moist cotton ball in place over eye until secretions softened.			
8. Once eye was clean, instilled liquid tear solution or Lacrilube ointment into the conjunctival sac of eye.			
9. Turned client's head to opposite side and repeated steps 6 through 8 for other eye.			
10. If eyes remained open, closed eye gently and covered with protective patch.			
11. Removed gloves and washed hands.			
12. Documented procedure correctly.			

Additional Comments:

_____

_____

_____

_____

_____

_____

_____

Name _____   Specific Skill Performed _____
Date _____   Attempt Number _____
Instructor _____   PASS _____   FAIL _____

PERFORMANCE CHECKLIST 10.4   **TAKING CARE OF ARTIFICIAL EYES**

	S	U	COMMENTS
1. Assessed client's usual method of cleaning.			
2. Washed hands and applied gloves.			
3. Assessed client's eyelids and socket.			
4. Explained procedure to client.			
5. Placed client in sitting or supine position.			
6. Lined labeled container with gauze and filled with water.			
7. Pulled down lower eyelid; exerted slight pressure below eyelid.			
8. Caught artificial eye in hand and placed in container.			
9. If artificial eye did not slide out, used small suction cup to remove eye.			
10. Washed artificial eye with saline or mild soap.			
11. Rinsed artificial eye with saline or under running water and dried thoroughly.			
12. Placed artificial eye in labeled container.			
13. Pulled down lower lid and cleaned eye socket by irrigating with warm water or saline.			
14. Washed and dried external eye wall.			
15. Reinserted prosthesis correctly.			
16. Removed gloves and washed hands.			
17. Placed client in position of comfort.			
18. Documented procedure correctly.			

Additional Comments:

_____

_____

_____

Name _____   Specific Skill Performed _____
Date _____   Attempt Number _____
Instructor _____   PASS _____   FAIL _____

PERFORMANCE CHECKLIST 10.5   TAKING CARE OF CONTACT LENSES

	S	U	COMMENTS
1. Assessed client's usual method of caring for contact lenses.			
2. Assessed client's self-care abilities.			
3. Assessed condition of eyes. If eye injury present, did not remove lenses.			
4. Explained procedure to client.			
Removing and Cleaning Lenses			
5. Raised bed to comfortable working level.			
6. Opened storage case noting which side is marked right and which is marked left.			
7. Washed hands and applied gloves.			
8. Checked to see if lenses are hard or soft.			
Removing Hard Lenses			
9. Centered lens over cornea, then gently spread eyelids apart.			
10. Held upper eyelid in place while pressing lower eyelid up under bottom rim of lens.			
11. Once lens loosened from cornea and began to tilt, moved eyelids toward each other.			
12. Caught lens in lower hand.			
Removing Soft Lenses			
13. Pulled down on lower eyelid and applied gentle pressure on upper eyelid to move lens partly onto sclera.			
14. Used pads of thumb and index finger of lower hand to grasp lens and remove it.			
15. Cleaned lens with cleaning solution and rinsed well.			

	S	U	COMMENTS
16. Placed lenses properly in storage case and covered with saline solution.			
17. Tightly closed lid of case, making sure lid not closed on lens.			
18. Assessed eyes for damage or irritation.			
19. Documented removal correctly.			

Inserting Lenses

	S	U	COMMENTS
20. Removed each lens from container and moistened with appropriate wetting solution.			
21. Observed lens for damage and correct appearance.			
22. Placed lens on index finger of your dominant hand.			
23. Held client's upper and lower eyelids open and asked client to look straight ahead.			
24. Placed lens directly over client's iris and pupil.			
25. Gently rubbed upper lid with finger to remove air bubbles.			
26. Assessed client's comfort. If necessary, removed, cleaned, and reinserted lens.			
27. Documented procedure correctly.			

Additional Comments:

_____

_____

_____

_____

_____

_____

_____

_____

_____

Name _____   Specific Skill Performed _____
Date _____   Attempt Number _____
Instructor _____   PASS _____   FAIL _____

PERFORMANCE CHECKLIST 10.6   IRRIGATING THE EARS

	S	U	COMMENTS
1. Assessed client's ear canal and pinna for redness, lesions, drainage, and pain.			
2. Explained procedure to client.			
3. Prepared solution in the proper amount and at the proper temperature.			
4. Washed hands and applied gloves.			
5. Cleaned outer ear and ear canal if necessary.			
6. Placed towel over client and under the ear to be irrigated.			
7. Turned client's head so that ear to be irrigated is facing downward.			
8. Placed emesis basin below client's ear and filled bulb syringe with solution.			
9. Pulled ear auricle up and back to straighten ear canal.			
10. Placed tip of bulb syringe inside client's ear canal and gently squeezed syringe to direct solution toward upper wall of ear canal.			
11. Dried client's outer ear and instructed client to lie on affected side for a period of time.			
12. Noted discharge obtained from ear then discarded solution appropriately.			
13. Cleaned and disposed of equipment properly.			
14. Removed gloves and washed hands.			
15. Reexamined client's ear.			
16. Documented procedure correctly.			

Additional Comments:

_____

_____

_____

PERFORMANCE CHECKLIST 10.7   **TAKING CARE OF A HEARING AID**

	S	U	COMMENTS
1. Assessed for number of hearing aids and usual method of care.			
2. Gently removed hearing aid and turned hearing aid off.			
3. Wiped aid with a dry tissue.			
4. Examined aid for wax plugs, cracks, and twisting of plastic tubing.			
5. Opened battery compartment of hearing aid and placed in storage case.			
6. Assessed for ear discomfort.			
7. Gently washed ear with clean washcloth and soap and water. Rinsed and dried ear.			
Insertion of Hearing Aid			
8. Closed battery compartment tightly and assessed that battery is working.			
9. Turned aid off and inserted into ear canal.			
10. Turned aid on and adjusted volume for client's hearing comfort.			
11. If feedback present, pressed in on earmold to check for looseness or need to reposition.			
12. Documented procedure correctly.			

Additional Comments:

_____

_____

_____

_____

_____

_____

_____

Name _____ Specific Skill Performed _____

Date _____ Attempt Number _____

Instructor _____ PASS _____ FAIL _____

PERFORMANCE CHECKLIST 10.8   GIVING A COMPLETE BED BATH

	S	U	COMMENTS
1. Checked orders and precautions for moving and positioning.			
2. Assessed self-care abilities and explained procedure to client.			
3. Assessed for tubes and IV lines to prevent their inadvertent removal.			
4. Gathered appropriate equipment and hygiene aids. Placed within reach.			
5. Adjusted room temperature and ventilation. Offered bedpan or urinal.			
6. Placed client in supine position if not contraindicated.			
7. Adjusted bed to comfortable working height with opposite side rail up.			
8. Washed hands and put on gloves.			
9. Removed top linen, covered with bath blanket. Removed client's gown.			
10. Filled bath basin 1/2 full with warm water. Obtained fresh water as needed.			
11. Removed pillow and placed bath towel under head.			
12. Folded washcloth into mitt and washed eyes without soap. Dried from inner to outer canthus.			
13. Washed, rinsed, and dried face, ears, and neck, and removed towel from under head.			
14. Placed towel lengthwise under far arm. Washed, rinsed, and dried arm and axillae. Repeated for near arm.			
15. Applied deodorant to axillae if desired.			
16. Placed far then near hand in water with bath towel under basin.			
17. Washed and dried each hand and all sides of each finger.			
18. Placed towel over chest and fan-folded bath blanket to umbilicus.			

	S	U	COMMENTS
19. Washed, rinsed, and dried chest correctly, applying dusting of talc under breasts if desired.			
20. Placed second towel over abdomen and fan-folded bath blanket to pubic region.			
21. Washed, rinsed, and dried each side of abdomen correctly.			
22. Repositioned bath blanket at shoulders and removed towels.			
23. Exposed far leg, sliding bath blanket toward center of hips. Placed towel lengthwise under leg.			
24. Securely positioned bath basin near foot to be bathed and with knee bent placed foot firmly in bath basin.			
25. Washed circumference of leg with mitted washcloth and foot with open washcloth.			
26. Dried leg and foot thoroughly paying special attention to area between toes.			
27. Follow steps 23 through 26 for near leg and foot.			
28. Turned client to side-lying position facing away from you keeping covered with bath blanket.			
29. Washed, rinsed, and dried back.			
30. Washed rinsed, and dried buttocks and perianal area.			
31. Helped client assume a supine position.			
32. Obtained fresh water and washed, rinsed, and dried perineal area.			
33. Removed and disposed of gloves, applied moisturizing lotion to client's skin.			
34. Assisted client with dressing and placed in position of comfort and safety with call light in reach.			
35. Disposed of soiled linen; cleaned and replaced equipment.			
36. Washed hands.			
37. Documented significant findings, condition of skin, and client's tolerance of procedure.			

Name _____   Specific Skill Performed _____
Date _____   Attempt Number _____
Instructor _____   PASS _____   FAIL _____

PERFORMANCE CHECKLIST 10.9   **PROVIDING HYGIENIC CARE OF THE GENITALIA FOR THE MALE CLIENT**

	S	U	COMMENTS
1. Assessed client's self-care abilities.			
2. Explained procedure to client.			
3. Provided opportunity to empty bladder and bowels.			
4. Washed hands and applied gloves.			
5. Provided privacy and draped client with bath blanket.			
6. Positioned bed at comfortable working height.			
7. Assessed genital area.			
8. Filled bath basin 1/2 full with warm water.			
9. Helped client spread his legs apart.			
10. Thoroughly washed penis and scrotum correctly.			
11. Rinsed and dried penis and scrotum well.			
12. Turned client on side and draped correctly.			
13. Washed, rinsed, and dried anal area correctly.			
14. Removed soiled linens and replaced top sheets.			
15. Lowered bed and placed client in position of comfort.			
16. Cleaned up area.			
17. Removed gloves and washed hands.			
18. Documented procedure correctly.			

Additional Comments:

_____

_____

_____

_____

Name _____   Specific Skill Performed _____
Date _____   Attempt Number _____
Instructor _____   PASS _____   FAIL _____

PERFORMANCE CHECKLIST 10.10 **PROVIDING HYGIENIC CARE OF THE GENITALIA**
FOR THE FEMALE CLIENT

	S	U	COMMENTS
1. Assessed client's self-care abilities.			
2. Explained procedure to client.			
3. Provided opportunity to empty bladder and bowels.			
4. Washed hands and applied gloves.			
5. Provided privacy and draped client with bath blanket.			
6. Positioned bed at comfortable working height.			
7. Assessed genital area.			
8. Filled irrigating bottle with warm soapy water or cleansing solution.			
9. Assisted client onto bedpan.			
10. Helped client spread her legs apart and separated labia with nondominant hand.			
11. Poured cleansing solution over genital area. If necessary, cleansed again with washcloth using correct procedure.			
12. Rinsed and dried genitalia gently.			
13. Removed bedpan and turned client to side.			
14. Cleansed, rinsed, and dried anal area correctly.			
15. Placed client in position of comfort.			
16. Removed soiled linens and replaced top sheets.			
17. Cleaned up area. Removed gloves and washed hands.			
18. Documented procedure correctly.			

Additional Comments:

_____

_____

Name _____   Specific Skill Performed _____
Date _____   Attempt Number _____
Instructor _____   PASS _____   FAIL _____

PERFORMANCE CHECKLIST 10.11 TAKING CARE OF THE HANDS

	S	U	COMMENTS
1. Explained procedure to client.			
2. Assessed condition of client's nails.			
3. Placed client in upright position.			
4. Protected bed linen with waterproof pads.			
5. Positioned bedside table covered with towel over client's lap.			
6. Filled basin 1/2 full with warm water and cleansing agent.			
7. Placed basin on overbed table.			
8. Soaked client's fingers in basin for 10 to 15 minutes.			
9. Applied gloves.			
10. Placed client's hands on towel and refilled basin.			
11. Rinsed client's hands and dried thoroughly.			
12. Gently cleaned under each fingernail with orange stick.			
13. Gently pushed each cuticle back using washcloth or rounded edges of orange stick.			
14. Cut nails correctly and smoothed edges with emery board.			
15. Massaged from fingertips to wrists with lotion.			
16. Assisted client to comfortable position.			
17. Cleaned up area.			
18. Removed gloves and washed hands.			
19. Documented procedure correctly.			

Additional Comments:

_____

_____

_____

Name _____   Specific Skill Performed _____

Date _____   Attempt Number _____

Instructor _____   PASS _____   FAIL _____

PERFORMANCE CHECKLIST 10.12 **PROVIDING FOOT CARE**

	S	U	COMMENTS
1. Assessed reason for foot care and underlying medical conditions.			
2. Explained procedure to client.			
3. Placed client in Fowler's position. Placed waterproof pad under feet.			
4. Filled basin 1/2 full with warm water and cleansing agent.			
5. Washed hands and applied gloves.			
6. Soaked client's feet in basin for 10 to 15 minutes.			
7. Rubbed calloused and dirty areas with a washcloth.			
8. Removed feet from water and placed them on a towel.			
9. Cleaned under toenails with orange stick.			
10. Filled basin with fresh water and rinsed feet well. Dried feet thoroughly.			
11. Trimmed client's toenails straight across with clippers.			
12. Smoothed rough edges with emery board.			
13. Massaged client's feet with lotion from heels to toes.			
14. Helped client to assume position of comfort.			
15. Cleaned up supplies.			
16. Removed gloves and washed hands.			
17. Documented procedure correctly.			

Additional Comments:

_____

_____

_____

_____

Name _____ Specific Skill Performed _____
Date _____ Attempt Number _____
Instructor _____ PASS _____   FAIL _____

PERFORMANCE CHECKLIST 10.13 **PROVIDING HAIR CARE**

	S	U	COMMENTS
1. Washed hands.			
2. Gathered proper and clean equipment.			
3. Explained procedure to client.			
4. Assessed condition of client's hair and scalp.			
Brushing and Combing the Hair			
5. Assisted client to sitting position with towel draped over shoulders.			
6. Divided hair into sections. Began at sides of client's head then moved to back.			
7. Removed tangles beginning with brush or comb at end of hair and working toward scalp. Applied water, vinegar, or hydrogen peroxide to help loosen tangles.			
8. Styled hair according to client's preference or need.			
Special Considerations for Clients With Very Curly Hair			
9. Divided hair into small sections and brushed to remove tangles.			
10. Combed hair working from ends to scalp.			
11. Applied oil or petroleum jelly to scalp if necessary.			
12. Used pick for styling.			
Hair Care for the Man With a Mustache and Beard			
13. Combed facial hair daily.			
14. Shampooed facial hair with mild shampoo.			

	S	U	COMMENTS
Shampooing Hair of Client in Bed			
15. Positioned bed at comfortable working height.			
16. Moved client to end of bed nearest you.			
17. Removed pillow. Placed plastic covered with towel under head and neck.			
18. Obtained plastic shampoo tray and positioned under client's head with drain end over side of bed.			
19. Placed bucket or basin close to bed to catch drainage.			
20. Placed washcloth over the client's eyes.			
21. Applied warm water until hair is thoroughly wet.			
22. Applied small amount of shampoo and worked into lather.			
23. Massaged all portions of scalp beginning at hairline and working toward back of head.			
24. Rinsed hair thoroughly. Applied conditioner if needed.			
25. Squeezed excess water from hair and wrapped head with bath towel.			
26. Used towel and hair dryer to dry scalp and hair thoroughly.			
27. Groomed and styled hair as desired.			
28. Placed dry clothing on client and made sure bed linens were dry.			
29. Lowered bed to safe height and positioned patient for comfort and safety.			
30. Cleaned area and properly disposed of equipment.			
31. Washed hands.			
32. Documented procedure correctly.			

Additional Comments:

_____

_____

_____

_____

Name _____   Specific Skill Performed _____
Date _____   Attempt Number _____
Instructor _____   PASS _____   FAIL _____

PERFORMANCE CHECKLIST 10.14 **SHAVING A CLIENT**

	S	U	COMMENTS
1. Assessed client's self-care abilities and proneness to bleed.			
2. Gathered appropriate supplies.			
3. Washed hands and applied gloves.			
4. Explained procedure to client.			
5. Assisted client to high-Fowler's or semi-Fowler's position.			
6. Placed towel over chest and around shoulders.			
7. Soaked area to be shaved with warm to hot washcloth until hair is soft.			
8. Applied lathered soap or shaving cream.			
9. Pulled skin taut on area to be shaved with nondominant hand and held razor at 45° angle.			
10. Moved razor in direction that hair grows using short, firm, gentle strokes and being careful not to cut the skin.			
11. Continued until all areas were shaved avoiding injured tissue areas, rinsing razor in between areas.			
12. After all areas were shaved, rinsed shaved area thoroughly with moistened warm washcloth.			
13. Dried area and applied after-shave or lotion as desired.			
14. Cleaned razor and disposed of blades in an appropriate container.			
15. Assisted client to position of comfort and safety.			
16. Washed hands.			
17. Documented procedure correctly.			

Additional Comments:

_____

_____

_____

Name _____   Specific Skill Performed _____
Date _____   Attempt Number _____
Instructor _____   PASS _____   FAIL _____

PERFORMANCE CHECKLIST 10.15 **BATHING AN INFANT**

	S	U	COMMENTS
1. Make sure room is warm and free of drafts.			
2. Washed hands and applied gloves.			
3. Filled basin or small tub with water at correct temperature.			
4. Washed each of infant's eyes with separate moist cotton ball from inner to outer canthus			
5. Washed external ear and behind ear with washcloth around your index finger.			
6. Washed face with washcloth and water only.			
7. Washed infant's neck using mild soap. Sat infant up while supporting neck and shoulders and dried thoroughly.			
8. Correctly held infant in football position with head over basin. Lathered scalp with mild soap or shampoo.			
9. Rinsed and dried scalp and hair thoroughly. Brushed hair with soft bristle brush.			
10. Placed infant in supine position and removed shirt and diaper. Wiped fecal material away from perineum or buttocks.			
11. Covered infant's body with clean dry towel.			
12. Washed infant's arms, axilla, chest, and abdomen with washcloth and soap.			
13. Rinsed and dried each body part thoroughly. Covered infant with towel.			
14. Cleaned umbilical area with soap and water without wetting the umbilical cord.			
15. Rinsed and dried umbilical area. Applied alcohol to umbilical cord stump.			
16. Exposed one leg and foot at a time. Washed, rinsed, and dried each leg and foot.			
17. Placed infant on stomach. Washed, rinsed, and dried back. Covered infant with towel.			

	S	U	COMMENTS
18. Applied lotion or ointment to dry skin areas.			
19. Placed infant in supine position and correctly washed genitalia and perineum.			
20. Lifted infant by ankles and washed, rinsed and dried buttocks. Applied jelly or ointment to anal area if needed.			
21. Applied clean diaper correctly.			
22. Dressed infant and bundled in a blanket.			
23. Placed infant in side-lying position in crib.			
24. Cleaned equipment properly and returned to storage area.			
25. Removed gloves and washed hands.			
26. Correctly documented procedure and infant's response.			
Giving a Tub Bath			
27. Followed steps 1 through 10 above.			
28. Slowly immersed infant feet first into tub of water.			
29. Positioned infant by supporting head and shoulders with your arm and holding thigh with your hand.			
30. Washed infant with soap and rinsed beginning with shoulders and moving down to lower extremities.			
31. Removed infant from tub and dried thoroughly. Wrapped infant in towel.			
32. Applied lotion or ointment to dry skin areas.			
33. Followed steps 21 through 26 above.			

Additional Comments:

_____

_____

_____

_____

_____

Name _____ Specific Skill Performed _____
Date _____ Attempt Number _____
Instructor _____ PASS _____   FAIL _____

PERFORMANCE CHECKLIST 10.16 MAKING AN UNOCCUPIED BED

	S	U	COMMENTS
1. Assessed client for movement limitations.			
2. Washed hands.			
3. Obtained clean linen needed.			
4. Assisted client to chair.			
5. Adjusted bed to comfortable working height and loosened all soiled linen from under mattress.			
6. Removed soiled linen and pillowcase and disposed of in appropriate linen hamper. Did not shake linens or allow them to come into contact with uniform.			
Changing the Bottom Linen			
7. Pulled mattress to head of bed. Wiped off and dried mattress as needed.			
8. Applied all clean linen to one side of bed before moving to other side.			
9. From side of bed, spread out mattress pad, and smoothed out wrinkles.			
10. Placed bottom sheet even with foot of bed and with center fold in middle of bed.			
11. Opened sheet lengthwise and fan-folded top layer to middle of bed.			
12. Correctly mitered corner at head of bed.			
13. Tucked bottom sheet securely under mattress.			
14. Placed draw sheet correctly over bottom sheet and tucked excess edge of draw sheet under mattress.			
15. Moved to opposite side of bed. Smoothed mattress pad and bottom sheet and correctly mitered corner at head of bed.			
16. Pulled bottom sheet tight using good body mechanics and tucked sheet under mattress.			

	S	U	COMMENTS
17. Smoothed draw sheet over bottom sheet, pulled draw sheet tight and tucked securely under mattress.			
Changing the Top Linen			
18. Placed top sheet and blanket on bed with center fold in middle of bed and top of sheet even with top of mattress.			
19. Correctly made toe pleat in top linen, tucked linen under foot of bed, and correctly mitered corner at foot of bed.			
20. Moved to opposite side of bed and smoothed out top linens.			
21. Leaving toe pleat in top linen, tucked linen under foot of bed and correctly mitered corner at foot of bed.			
22. Correctly applied pillowcase to pillow and placed in center at head of bed with open end away from door.			
23. Made cuff at top edge of top linen and fan-folded to foot of bed.			
24. Attached call light to bed and returned bed to low position.			
25. Assisted client back to bed, if desired, and placed in position of comfort and safety.			
26. Placed client's needed items within easy reach.			
27. Properly discarded soiled linens.			
28. Washed hands.			

Additional Comments:

_____

_____

_____

_____

_____

_____

_____

_____

Name _____   Specific Skill Performed _____
Date _____   Attempt Number _____
Instructor _____   PASS _____   FAIL _____

PERFORMANCE CHECKLIST 10.17 **MAKING AN OCCUPIED BED**

	S	U	COMMENTS
1. Assessed client for movement limitations.			
2. Obtained appropriate supplies. Placed within easy reach.			
3. Explained procedure to client, adjusted bed to comfortable working height and lowered proximal side rail.			
4. Removed top linen except for loosened top sheet or bath blanket.			
5. Folded soiled linens and disposed of correctly to prevent spread of microorganisms.			
6. Positioned client on far side of bed, facing away from you in side-lying position.			
Changing the Bottom Linen			
7. Loosened bottom linens and fan-folded to middle of bed tucking under client's shoulder, back, and buttocks.			
8. If mattress pad is to be changed, fan-folded to middle of bed. If not, smoothed out wrinkles.			
9. Wiped off and dried mattress if needed.			
10. Applied all clean linen to one side before moving to other side.			
11. Placed clean bottom sheet even with foot of bed with center fold in middle of bed.			
12. Opened sheet lengthwise and fan-folded top layer to middle of bed tucking under soiled sheet.			
13. Tucked bottom sheet under mattress at head of bed and correctly mitered corner.			
14. Faced side of bed and tucked side edge of sheet under mattress.			
15. Placed draw sheet over bottom sheet correctly.			
16. Laid center fold of draw sheet along middle of bed. Fan-folded top layer toward client tucking under client and soiled sheets.			
17. Tucked outer edges of draw sheet under mattress.			

	S	U	COMMENTS
18. Warned client of lump in bed and assisted client to roll onto side facing you.			
19. Raised side rail on side client is facing and moved to other side of bed. Lowered side rail.			
20. Removed soiled linen rolling soiled areas to inside. Disposed of properly.			
21. Wiped off and dried mattress.			
22. Smoothed fan-folded clean linen to edge of bed.			
23. Repositioned client in supine position and pulled bottom linens toward you to smooth out wrinkles.			
24. Tucked bottom sheet under mattress at head of bed and correctly mitered corner.			
25. Leaned back and pulled down to tuck excess linen under mattress.			
26. Leaned back and pulled down on draw sheet then tucked middle, upper, and lower draw sheet under mattress.			

Changing the Top Linen

	S	U	COMMENTS
27. Placed clean top sheet over client with center fold in middle of bed and unfolded sheet across client.			
28. Asked client to hold clean top sheet, moved to foot of bed, pulled out soiled top sheet and blanket, rolling into bundle as you pulled.			
29. Placed blanket over client if needed and tucked top linens under mattress foot. Correctly mitered corners.			
30. Loosened top linens at toes and raised head of bed as needed for comfort.			
31. Removed soiled pillowcase. Applied clean pillowcase to pillow correctly.			
32. Supported client's head while placing pillow under head with closed end of pillowcase toward door.			
33. Placed client in position of comfort with call light in reach.			
34. Disposed of soiled linen properly.			
35. Washed hands.			

Name _____   Specific Skill Performed _____

Date _____   Attempt Number _____

Instructor _____   PASS _____   FAIL _____

PERFORMANCE CHECKLIST 10.18 MAKING A SURGICAL BED

	S	U	COMMENTS
1. Washed hands.			
2. Determined necessity for making surgical bed.			
3. Prepared bed as indicated for unoccupied bed.			
4. Left pillow off bed but in easily accessible place.			
5. Placed draw sheet and incontinence pads appropriately over bottom sheet.			
6. Tucked in excess draw sheet at sides of mattress.			
7. Fan-folded top covers to bottom or side of mattress.			
8. Left bed in high position with side rails down.			
9. Disposed of soiled linens in proper area.			
10. Placed IV pole at head of bed.			
11. Placed tissues, an emesis basin, a towel and washcloth at bedside.			
12. Positioned furniture to allow for passage of stretcher.			
13. Washed hands.			

Additional Comments:

_____

_____

_____

_____

_____

_____

_____

_____

_____

Name _____   Specific Skill Performed _____

Date _____   Attempt Number _____

Instructor _____   PASS _____   FAIL _____

PERFORMANCE CHECKLIST 11.1   GIVING A BACK RUB (BACK MASSAGE)

	S	U	COMMENTS
1. Assessed for presence of contraindications and limitations to positioning.			
2. Explained procedure to client.			
3. Allowed client to empty bladder and complete other hygiene measures.			
4. Washed hands.			
5. Adjusted bed to working height.			
6. Positioned client in prone position with back, shoulders, upper arms, and buttocks exposed and rest of body covered with bath blanket. Used side-lying position if prone not allowed.			
7. Warmed hands and obtained lubricant, rubbed lubricant between hands.			
8. Gently applied lubricant to sacral area stroking from base of buttocks up to shoulders, over upper arms, and back to base of buttocks using smooth, firm, even strokes.			
9. Kept palmar surface of both hands parallel to spine and in contact with the skin at all times.			
10. Correctly kneaded 1/2 of back and upper arm starting at buttocks and moving up to shoulder, deltoid and upper arm, and returning to buttocks.			
11. Repeated kneading on other side of body.			
12. Used friction correctly over back by exerting pressure in a small circular motion around but not over bony prominences.			
13. Rhythmically proceeded from stroking to kneading to friction, reapplying lubricant as needed.			
14. Ended massage with long, stroking movements, gradually decreasing pressure until massage completed.			
15. Wiped excess lubricant from client's back with towel.			
16. For side-lying position, massaged upper side then turned patient to massage other side.			

	S	U	COMMENTS
17. Covered client and placed in position of comfort and safety.			
18. Washed hands.			
19. Documented massage and condition of skin.			

Additional Comments:

_____

_____

_____

_____

_____

_____

_____

_____

_____

_____

_____

_____

_____

Name _____ Specific Skill Performed _____

Date _____ Attempt Number _____

Instructor _____ PASS _____ FAIL _____

PERFORMANCE CHECKLIST 12.1   GIVING A SITZ BATH

	S	U	COMMENTS
1. Checked client's chart for order/rationale/contraindications to sitz bath.			
2. Discussed procedure with client. Explained what to expect during and following the procedure.			
3. Washed hands.			
4. Prepared sitz bath: a. Unit sitz bath: cleaned with disinfectant, rinsed well and placed clean towels around rim. b. Portable sitz bath: placed bowl on toilet and followed manufacturer's instruction for setup.			
5. Filled sitz bath bowl 1/3 to 1/2 full with water (100° to 105°F).			
6. Assisted client to undress and immerse perineum in sitz bath. Draped client appropriately for warmth and privacy.			
7. Assessed client comfort and provided emergency call light for client use.			
8. Instructed/allowed client to remain in sitz bath for 15 to 20 minutes.			
9. Checked client frequently. Refilled sitz bath as needed to keep water temperature warm.			
10. When sitz bath finished, assisted client as needed (i.e., drying off, re-dress, etc.). Used gloves if appropriate.			
11. Assisted client to bed and performed appropriate assessments (i.e., comfort, changes in perineum, etc.).			
12. Emptied and cleaned sitz bath. Disposed of towels and gloves appropriately.			
13. Washed hands.			
14. Documented procedure including assessment data and client tolerance of sitz bath.			

Additional Comments:

_____

Name _____ Specific Skill Performed _____

Date _____ Attempt Number _____

Instructor _____ PASS _____ FAIL _____

PERFORMANCE CHECKLIST 12.2 **TEACHING PROGRESSIVE MUSCLE RELAXATION**

	S	U	COMMENTS
1. Determined nature of client illness.			
2. Asked client to wear comfortable clothes and to empty his/her bladder.			
3. Provided quiet environment and asked client to assume a comfortable position (i.e., bed or chair).			
4. Asked client to close his/her eyes and focus on a muscle group (i.e., muscles in lower arms and hands). Asked client to: a. Consciously tense the muscles and note the sensation of tenseness b. Hold the tenseness for 5 to 7 seconds c. Relax the muscles and concentrate on the differences in sensations (i.e., tenseness vs. relaxation)			
5. Asked client to duplicate the procedure with other major muscle groups throughout body. Had client start with upper body and work downward.			
6. Had client breathe slowly, deeply, and rhythmically while practicing PMR unless contraindicated (i.e., respiratory problems). Discouraged hyperventilation.			
7. Encouraged client to continue PMR for 15 to 20 seconds.			
8. At end of exercise, encouraged client to: a. Concentrate on rhythmic breathing for 1 minute b. Open eyes slowly c. Stretch (i.e., as if awakening from sleep) d. Move around until he/she feels alert			
9. Instructed client to practice PMR exercises at least 2 x day for 15 to 20 minutes.			
10. Encouraged client progress. Encouraged client to ignore distracting thoughts during practice.			
11. Provided audiotape if needed to assist client mastery of technique.			
12. Recorded the procedure and relevant information including evaluation of client response.			

Name _____   Specific Skill Performed _____

Date _____   Attempt Number _____

Instructor _____   PASS _____   FAIL _____

PERFORMANCE CHECKLIST 12.3   MONITORING A PATIENT-CONTROLLED ANALGESIA PUMP

	S	U	COMMENTS
1. Checked physician's orders for drug, dosage, administration parameters, and rationale.			
2. Assessed client's knowledge about procedure/rationale. Explained/instructed client/family regarding operation and expectations.			
3. Assessed client for level of consciousness and other pertinent data.			
4. Assessed IV site and patency. Ensured that primary IV was correct solution and infusing at proper rate as ordered.			
5. Checked client's ID band before preparing medication and again before beginning the administration.			
6. Obtained the PCA pump/tubing and prepared the medication.			
7. Properly placed the medication/syringe infusion inside the pump and flushed the tubing.			
8. Checked client's ID again before connecting PCA tubing to primary IV line (18-gauge needle/injection port). Secured all connections.			
9. Set all medication dials to lowest settings.			
10. Followed manufacturer's setup instructions for pump. Followed physician's/agency standing orders regarding dosing parameters.			
11. After administering loading dose, gave client the "button" for self-administration. Checked to be sure he/she knew how to operate it.			
12. Frequently evaluated client's condition and patency of IV and PCA system (i.e., per agency protocol, as ordered, as needed):			
13. Followed manufacturer's instructions for continued operation of pump (i.e., replacing syringe, obtaining administration history/amount infused, alarms, etc.).			
14. Recorded the procedure appropriately (chart, narcotic records, etc.).			

Name _____   Specific Skill Performed _____
Date _____   Attempt Number _____
Instructor _____   PASS _____   FAIL _____

PERFORMANCE CHECKLIST 12.4   APPLYING MOIST HEAT

	S	U	COMMENTS
1. Checked the client's chart for physician's order, rationale and possible contraindications (i.e., impaired sensation) for application of moist heat.			
2. Discussed procedure with client. Explained rationale and what to expect, including necessity for sterile technique if appropriate.			
3. Gathered appropriate equipment/supplies.			
4. Washed hands.			
5. Warmed container of solution (i.e., sterile saline or tap water) to appropriate temperature in basin filled with hot water. Followed manufacturer's instructions to heat commercial compresses.			
6. Place waterproof pad under affected area.			
7. Put thin layer of petroleum jelly on client's skin if appropriate.			
8. Poured sterile solution into sterile basin. Soaked appropriate compresses in solution (i.e., 4 x 4s, towel, etc.), wrung out excess liquid and placed on affected area. Used sterile gloves/sterile technique if appropriate.			
9. Wrapped area with waterproof pad or applied disposable heat pack or aquathermia pad.			
10. Checked client's skin periodically for heat intolerance.			
11. Left compress in place 20 minutes if tolerated.			
12. Removed compress and dried area.			
13. Disposed of soiled equipment appropriately.			
14. Washed hands.			
15. Reassessed client's skin.			
16. Documented the procedure including assessment data and client response.			

Name _____   Specific Skill Performed _____

Date _____   Attempt Number _____

Instructor _____   PASS _____   FAIL _____

PERFORMANCE CHECKLIST 12.5   **APPLYING DRY HEAT**

	S	U	COMMENTS
1. Checked the client's chart for physician's order, diagnosis, rationale, and possible contraindications (i.e., impaired sensation, sedation, agitation, inability to cooperate, presence of diabetes, etc.) for application of dry heat.			
2. Gathered appropriate equipment, discussed procedure with client, and assessed affected area.			
3. If using hot water bottle: a. Adjusted heated tap water to appropriate temperature. b. Filled hot water bottle 2/3 full. Expelled air. Checked for leaks. c. Wrapped bottle in protective cover and placed on affected area.			
4. If using disposable heat pack: a. Activated pack according to directions. b. Put pack in protective cover and placed it on affected area. c. Discarded pack after use.			
5. If using heating pad: a. Covered heating pad with protective cover (i.e., flannel). b. Cautioned client not to lie on heating pad or increase heating level. c. Turned switch to low. Placed heating pad on affected area.			
6. If using aquathermia pad: a. Prepared control unit according to manufacturer's directions. b. Turned unit on and checked temperature of heated solution before applying pad to client. c. Checked unit, pad, and tubing for leaks. d. Placed towel around affected area, applied aquathermia pad and secured it with tape.			
7. Periodically checked client's skin for heat intolerance.			
8. Left pad in place for 20 minutes, then removed it.			
9. Returned equipment to appropriate place after dry heat application(s) are discontinued.			
10. Documented the procedure including assessment data and client response.			

Name _____   Specific Skill Performed _____
Date _____   Attempt Number _____
Instructor _____   PASS _____   FAIL _____

PERFORMANCE CHECKLIST 12.6 · **APPLYING COLD**

	S	U	COMMENTS
1. Checked client's chart for physician's order, diagnosis, rationale, and possible contraindications for cold therapy (i.e., circulatory impairment).			
2. Discussed procedure with client. Explained rationale and what to expect.			
3. Assessed affected site.			
4. Obtained appropriate equipment.			
5. If using an ice bag: 　a. Filled bag 3/4 full with ice. Expelled air. Checked for leaks. 　b. Wrapped bag with towel/cover and placed on affected area.			
6. If using an ice collar: 　a. Filled collar 3/4 full with ice. Expelled air. Checked for leaks. 　b. Wrapped collar with protective covering and placed around client's neck.			
7. If using a disposable cold pack: 　a. Activated pack according to manufacturer's directions. 　b. Wrapped pack with towel/cover and placed on affected area. 　c. Discarded pack after treatment.			
8. Periodically assessed client's skin for signs of cold intolerance.			
9. Left cold application in place for 30 minutes and then removed it.			
10. Reassessed condition of client's skin.			
11. Documented procedure in client's record including assessment data and client response.			

Additional Comments:

_____

_____

_____

_____

PERFORMANCE CHECKLIST 12.7   GIVING A TEPID SPONGE BATH

	S	U	COMMENTS
1. Assessed client condition to determine need and to collect data.			
2. Reviewed agency protocol regarding administration of tepid sponge baths. Obtained order if needed.			
3. Explained procedure to client/family.			
4. Gathered appropriate equipment.			
5. Raised bed, washed hands, and put on gloves.			
6. Removed client's clothing, covered him/her with bath blanket and placed waterproof pads underneath.			

7. If sponging with tepid water:
   a. Filled basin with tepid water. Moistened washcloths and placed compresses on client's forehead, groin, and axilla for 20 to 30 minutes.
   b. Sponged client's face and each extremity for 5 minutes. Turned client and sponged back and buttocks for 5 to 10 minutes.
   Dried client with towel after sponging.			

8. If giving a tepid tub bath: a. Immersed client into tepid tub water for 20 to 30 minutes. Supported client's head and shoulders.			
9. Monitored client's responses to treatment (i.e., vs q 10 minutes).			
10. Stopped bath when client's temperature is slightly above normal.			
11. Replaced client's clothing, covered him/her with a sheet, and replaced soiled linen and removed equipment.			
12. Positioned client for comfort, lowered bed, and removed gloves and washed hands.			
13. Documented the procedure including assessment data and client response.			
14. Monitored client's vital signs q 1 to 2 hours until stable.			

Name _____   Specific Skill Performed _____

Date _____   Attempt Number _____

Instructor _____   PASS _____   FAIL _____

PERFORMANCE CHECKLIST 12.8   USING A HYPOTHERMIA OR HYPERTHEMIA BLANKET

	S	U	COMMENTS
1. Assessed client (i.e., T, P, R) to determine need.			
2. Checked physician's orders regarding application and desired temperature.			
3. Discussed procedure with client/family. Explained rationale and what to expect.			
4. Obtained machine and followed manufacturer's directions for setup.			
5. Ensured that machine was in good operating condition (i.e., cord/plug not frayed, grounded, etc.)			
6. Placed blanket on bed between client and mattress and covered it with a sheet.			
7. Inserted temperature probe and taped to client's buttocks.			
8. Set machine to desired temperature and turned it on. Checked for leaks.			
9. Checked client's temperature every 15 minutes and turned machine off when client's temp approached desired level.			
10. Periodically checked client's temp with glass thermometer.			
11. Checked client's vital signs q 30 minutes and observed for shivering.			
12. Turned client q 1 to 2 hours and assessed skin.			
13. Documented the procedure including assessment data, client response, and treatment time.			

Additional Comments:

_____

_____

_____

_____

Name _____

Date _____

Instructor _____

Specific Skill Performed _____

Attempt Number _____

PASS _____   FAIL _____

PERFORMANCE CHECKLIST 13.1   ADMINISTERING WHOLE BLOOD AND PACKED RED BLOOD CELLS

	S	U	COMMENTS
1. Assessed order, reason for transfusion and client's history of prior transfusions.			
2. Explained procedure to client and obtained informed consent if required. Obtained baseline vital signs.			
3. Obtained and properly identified blood in laboratory. Checked the cross-match slip with a licensed person on the unit. Checked blood with client's armband.			
4. If administering whole blood, gently inverted bag several times to mix blood.			
5. Washed hands and applied gloves.			
Administering Whole Blood With Y-tubing			
6. Closed clamps on Y-tubing and inserted one spike into normal saline.			
7. Primed tubing, including spike for blood, with normal saline to remove air. Inserted free spike into blood bag.			
8. If IV line in place, assessed site for patency. If no IV in place, performed venipuncture (see Performance Checklist 19.1).			
9. Started infusion with normal saline and assessed patency of IV.			
10. Started infusion of blood at keep-open rate for first 15 minutes and assessed client for signs of reaction.			
11. If no signs of reaction after 15 minutes, increased flow to prescribed rate.			
Administering Whole Blood or Packed Red Blood Cells With a Straight Blood Administration Set			
12. Ensured that an IV of normal saline is infusing and is patent.			
13. Inserted spike into port on blood product and filled drip chamber half-way.			

	S	U	COMMENTS
14. Placed 18-gauge needle on distal end of IV tubing and primed tubing with blood.			
15. Piggy-backed blood into most proximal port on IV tubing and secured with tape. Removed gloves.			
16. Repeated steps 10 and 11 above.			
17. Assessed client for blood reaction every 15 minutes for first hour, then every 30 minutes until infusion is complete.			
18. After infusion completed, flushed IV tubing with normal saline.			
19. Applied gloves to disconnect blood bag from tubing.			
20. Disposed of used supplies and blood bag correctly.			
21. Completed cross-match slip and distributed copies correctly.			
22. Documented procedure and client's response correctly.			

Additional Comments:

_____

_____

_____

_____

_____

_____

_____

_____

_____

_____

_____

_____

_____

_____

_____

Name _____   Specific Skill Performed _____
Date _____   Attempt Number _____
Instructor _____   PASS _____   FAIL _____

PERFORMANCE CHECKLIST 13.1A   USING BLOOD-WARMING DEVICES

	S	U	COMMENTS
1. Plugged in blood-warming device			
2. Followed steps 1 through 7 from Performance Checklist 13.1. Prepared blood product using the correct infusion set for the type of warming device.			
3. Flushed the line with normal saline to remove air.			
To Use Boood-Warming Coil			
4. Turned on machine. Removed coil from wrapper and closed clamps.			
5. Attached male adapter on blood line to female adapter on blood-warming coil. Attached 18-gauge needle to distal end of coil.			
6. Immersed coil in basin with 98.6° water. Opened clamp and allowed blood to fill tubing.			
7. Proceeded with straight-line administration of blood product.			
8. Replace blood-warming coil after 24 hours.			
To Use Dry-heat Warmer			
9. Inserted warming bag into blood warmer. Attached bottom and top leads correctly,			
10. Secured warming bag correctly on support pins and secured pins.			
11. Closed blood warmer, secured latch, and turned on dry-heat warmer.			
12. Allowed blood to warm to proper temperature, then opened clamp to saline line allowing blood-warming bag to fill with saline.			
13. When saline in top lead chamber, closed main flow clamp and released chamber.			
14. Removed adapter cover and opened top lead. Opened clamp to expel air from line.			
15. Proceeded to administer blood product as with Y-set.			

	S	U	COMMENTS
Administering Blood Using a Pressure Cuff or Positive-Pressure Set			
16. Placed blood unit into pressure cuff correctly and hung on IV pole.			
17. Turned screw on pressure cuff counter clockwise. Compressed bulb to inflate cuff to correct pressure.			
18. Turned screw to maintain pressure and checked pressure frequently.			
19. When using a positive-pressure administration set, opened flow clamps and compressed and released pump chamber to pump blood into client. Allowed chamber to completely fill before compressing again.			

Additional Comments:

_____

_____

_____

_____

_____

_____

_____

_____

_____

_____

_____

_____

_____

_____

_____

Name _____   Specific Skill Performed _____
Date _____   Attempt Number _____
Instructor _____   PASS _____   FAIL _____

PERFORMANCE CHECKLIST 13.2   **ADMINISTERING PLATELETS AND FRESH FROZEN PLASMA**

	S	U	COMMENTS
1. Reviewed physician's order and client's transfusion history.			
2. Explained procedure to client and obtained signed consent form, if necessary. Obtained baseline vital signs.			
Administering Fresh Frozen Plasma With a Blood Administration Set			
3. Obtained blood product from blood bank and checked for right blood product and right patient.			
4. Washed hands and applied gloves.			
5. Assessed existing IV line for patency or performed venipuncture with needle of appropriate size. Used normal saline for infusion.			
6. Spiked plasma bag with blood administration set tubing. Attached needle to other end of tubing.			
7. Primed tubing with plasma to remove air.			
8. Used alcohol swab to cleanse port most proximal to insertion site on existing IV line.			
9. Closed clamp on saline infusion and adjusted clamp on the plasma to allow plasma to infuse at prescribed rate.			
Administering Platelets With a Component Drip Set			
10. Closed clamp on the administration set, pulled back tabs on the bag of platelets to open port, inserted spike into the port.			
11. Compressed drip chamber so that platelets covered the filter and attached needle to other end of tubing.			
12. Primed tubing with platelets to remove air.			
13. Used alcohol swab to cleanse port most proximal to insertion site on existing IV line.			
14. Closed clamp on saline infusion and opened clamp on platelets to allow platelets to flow in over 10 minutes.			

	S	U	COMMENTS
15. After platelets infused, restarted normal saline to flush IV line.			
16. Restarted original IV solution and adjusted flow to prescribed rate.			
17. Recorded procedure and patient's response correctly.			

Additional Comments:

_____

_____

_____

_____

_____

_____

_____

_____

_____

_____

PERFORMANCE CHECKLIST 13.3   **ADMINISTERING AUTOTRANSFUSION THERAPY**

	S	U	COMMENTS
1. Reviewed physician's orders and pertinent laboratory data.			
2. Explained procedure to client and washed hands.			
3. Assessed vital signs and any bleeding. Applied gloves.			
4. Correctly injected anticoagulant into injection port on line attached to yellow port.			
5. Hung Solcotrans unit on bed rail with yellow end up making certain correct clamps are open and recording proper information.			
6. Left red clamp open for gravity drainage or connected suction correctly.			
7. Assessed for continuous drainage in unit, and client's response.			
8. Gently agitated Solcotrans unit periodically.			
9. After unit filled, closed red and yellow slide clamps and compressed evacuator tube.			
10. Disconnected evacuator tube and red slide clamp correctly.			
11. Instilled anticoagulant correctly if further collection is desired. If no further collection, attached evacuator tube to sleeve connector correctly.			
Performing Reinfusion			
12. Reviewed physician's order.			
13. Positioned container with yellow cap in upward position.			
14. Washed hands and applied gloves.			
15. Removed white injection port connector and evacuator tube from yellow port.			
16. Inserted proper filter into yellow port and attached blood infusion set to tubing.			
17. Opened yellow slide clamp and removed white luer-lock protector.			

	S	U	COMMENTS
18. Applied pressure with hand bulb attached to white luer connector.			
19. Inverted container on IV pole correctly.			
20. Reinfused client's blood either by gravity or using pressure.			
21. Correctly and thoroughly monitored and recorded client's response to transfusion.			

Additional Comments:

_____

_____

_____

_____

_____

_____

_____

_____

_____

_____

_____

_____

_____

_____

_____

_____

Name _____

Date _____

Instructor _____

Specific Skill Performed _____

Attempt Number _____

PASS _____   FAIL _____

PERFORMANCE CHECKLIST 14.1   BOTTLE-FEEDING THE INFANT

	S	U	COMMENTS
1. Checked physician's order for type and amount of feeding.			
2. Assessed infant's usual feeding pattern and parents' experience with bottle-feeding.			
3. Washed hands.			
4. Assessed temperature of formula.			
5. Held infant correctly and placed bib under infant's chin.			
6. Inserted bottle nipple correctly into infant's mouth with bottle at 45° angle.			
7. Observed infant for respiratory distress or problems with feeding.			
8. Burped infant correctly about halfway through the feeding.			
9. Continued feeding infant until bottle empty, or infant stops sucking or falls asleep.			
10. Burped infant correctly after feeding.			
11. Checked to see if diaper needs changing.			
12. Returned infant to crib, placed infant on his/her side, and raised side rails.			
13. Documented amount and type of feeding and infant's response.			

Additional Comments:

_____

_____

_____

_____

_____

_____

_____

Name _____   Specific Skill Performed _____
Date _____   Attempt Number _____
Instructor _____   PASS _____   FAIL _____

PERFORMANCE CHECKLIST 14.2   **ASSISTING WITH BREAST-FEEDING**

	S	U	COMMENTS
1. Changed infant's diaper if necessary.			
2. Assessed mother's experience and knowledge related to breast feeding.			
3. Placed mother in position of comfort with breast accessible.			
4. Positioned infant correctly for grasping the mother's nipple.			
5. Helped infant to grasp the mother's nipple properly.			
6. Allowed infant to suck on first breast for 10 to 15 minutes.			
7. Helped mother to break infant's suction correctly.			
8. Instructed mother to burp infant between feedings from each breast.			
9. Repositioned mother and baby to allow feeding from second breast.			
10. Instructed mother to burp infant again after feeding.			
11. Checked diaper for soiling and change if necessary.			
12. Positioned infant on his/her side.			
13. Instructed mother to expose nipples to air to allow drying of breast milk.			
14. Encouraged mother to rest between feedings.			
15. Documented breast-feeding correctly.			

Additional Comments:

_____

_____

_____

_____

_____

_____

Name _____   Specific Skill Performed _____

Date _____   Attempt Number _____

Instructor _____   PASS _____   FAIL _____

PERFORMANCE CHECKLIST 14.3   **HELPING THE ADULT TO EAT**

	S	U	COMMENTS
1. Assessed client for self-care abilities and presence of gag reflex.			
2. Checked for correct diet, presence of food allergies, and preferences.			
3. Prepared atmosphere conducive to eating and explained to client that mealtime is near.			
4. Assisted client to chair or adjusted bed to sitting position.			
5. Assisted client with handwashing and oral hygiene, put false teeth, glasses and hearing aid in place if necessary.			
6. Washed hands.			
7. Placed tray within easy reach on overbed table and removed food covers.			
8. Encouraged client's independence as much as possible. Assisted in preparation only as needed.			
9. If visually impaired, told client where food is on plate according to clock face.			
10. If client needed to be fed, offered foods according to client preferences and in manageable bites.			
11. Made sure hot foods not too hot and cold foods are served cold.			
12. Placed one spoonful or forkful at a time above client's tongue.			
13. Provided relaxed atmosphere, allowing sufficient time for chewing and swallowing before offering another bite.			
14. Provided straw for drinks if necessary. Used napkin to wipe spills from client's face.			
15. Provided conversation and client education as appropriate during meal.			
16. Patiently continued to offer food until client indicates that he/she is finished.			
17. Removed tray, cleaned up spills, and changed soiled linen.			

	S	U	COMMENTS
18. Assisted client to wash hands and perform mouth care if desired.			
19. Placed client in position of comfort and safety.			
20. Documented amount eaten and tolerance of meal.			

Additional Comments:

_____

_____

_____

_____

_____

_____

_____

_____

_____

_____

_____

_____

_____

_____

PERFORMANCE CHECKLIST 14.4   HELPING THE CHILD TO EAT

	S	U	COMMENTS
1. Assessed child's developmental level.			
2. Washed your hands.			
3. Washed child's face and hands.			
4. Placed food and drinks in unbreakable containers.			
5. Placed child in upright position unless contraindicated and placed bib around child's neck.			
6. Made sure environment is relaxed and free of distractions.			
7. Offered food beginning with less sweet items and giving sweet item last.			
8. Placed food in child's mouth above tongue.			
9. Wiped spit-out food off with spoon and placed back in child's mouth.			
10. Talked to child while feeding.			
11. Fed child until food gone or child seems satisfied.			
12. When meal finished, washed child's hands and mouth.			
13. Documented amount and types of food eaten.			

Additional Comments:

_____

_____

_____

_____

_____

_____

_____

Name _____ Specific Skill Performed _____

Date _____ Attempt Number _____

Instructor _____ PASS _____   FAIL _____

PERFORMANCE CHECKLIST 14.5   INSERTING A NASOGASTRIC TUBE

	S	U	COMMENTS
1. Checked physician's order, client diagnosis, and purpose of tube.			
2. Assessed client's level of consciousness and ability to follow directions. Obtained assistance if needed.			
3. Explained procedure to client.			
4. Washed hands and applied gloves.			
5. Gathered correct equipment, checked that suction equipment works properly, and prepared tube properly.			
6. Adjusted height of bed to position of comfort and obtained proper lighting.			
7. Placed client in high Fowler's position with client's head tilted back if possible.			
8. Provided privacy, draped client's chest, placed tissues, and emesis basin within easy reach of client.			
9. Stood on appropriate side of client for handedness.			
10. Assessed patency of nares and chose unobstructed side for tube insertion.			
11. Measured tube correctly, marked tube for proper length, and found natural downward curve of tube.			
12. Applied gloves.			
13. Applied topical anesthetic jelly with cotton-tipped swab to inside of selected naris.			
14. Lubricated first 10 cm. (4 inches) of tube with water-soluable jelly.			
15. Inserted guidewire in flexible feeding tube.			
16. Gently inserted tube into naris following natural curve of tube. Advanced tube to nasopharynx.			
17. Instructed client to flex neck slightly, take sips of water through a straw, and swallow on command.			

	S	U	COMMENTS
18. As client swallowed, advanced tube measured distance. Stopped procedure and notified physician if obstruction noted.			
19. If client gagged or respiratory distress occurred, pulled tube back into oropharynx and allowed client to rest a few minutes before proceeding.			
20. Checked placement of tube correctly using at least two methods.			
21. For intestinal intubation, taped in a manner which allowed tube to advanced over a number of hours to small intestine.			
22. For intestinal intubation, checked placement with chest x-ray.			
23. Once tube is in prescribed position, anchored tube securely to clean, dry skin using nonallergenic tape and attached to gown for added security.			
24. Connected to suction or feedings as ordered.			
25. Administered oral hygiene and cleansed nostrils.			
26. Placed client in position of comfort and safety.			
27. Disposed of equipment appropriately.			
28. Washed hands.			
29. Documented placement of tube and tolerance of procedure.			

Additional Comments:

_____

_____

_____

_____

_____

_____

_____

_____

_____

Name _____   Specific Skill Performed _____
Date _____   Attempt Number _____
Instructor _____   PASS _____   FAIL _____

PERFORMANCE CHECKLIST 14.6   **COLLECTING A GASTRIC SPECIMEN**

	S	U	COMMENTS
1. Assessed need for gastric specimen.			
2. Explained procedure and placed client in Fowler's position.			
3. Gathered appropriate equipment.			
4. Washed hands and applied gloves.			
5. Inserted nasogastric tube if not already in place (refer to Performance Checklist 14.5).			
6. Withdrew 10 ml. of gastric secretions and disposed of in emesis basin. Assessed color and presence of blood.			
Assessing the pH of Gastric Contents			
7. Applied 1 drop of gastric secretions to pH test paper and waited 30 seconds.			
8. Determined results by comparing pH paper with color chart.			
Assessing for Presence of Occult Blood			
9. Applied 1 drop of gastric contents to occult blood test paper.			
10. Applied 2 drops of guiac developer over sample and 1 drop between positive and negative control monitors.			
11. Waited 60 seconds. Compared color to control monitors.			
Final Activities			
12. Reconnected nasogastric tube to suction or clamp if necessary. Withdrew tube if inserted only for specimen.			
13. Disposed of soiled equipment in an appropriate manner. Removed gloves and washed hands.			
14. Explained results to client. Helped client to assume position of comfort and offered mouth care.			
15. Documented procedure correctly.			

PERFORMANCE CHECKLIST 14.7   REMOVING A NASOGASTRIC TUBE

	S	U	COMMENTS
1. Checked physician's order and applied gloves.			
2. Placed client in high Fowler's position and placed drape across client's chest.			
3. Discontinued suction or feeding. Clamped tube and removed tape.			
4. Placed emesis basin near client.			
5. Instructed client to take a deep breath and hold it. Pulled out tube in one continuous motion and wrapped in drape.			
6. Removed gloves and washed hands.			
7. Gave oral and nasal hygiene.			
8. Documented removal of tube.			

Additional Comments:

_____

_____

_____

_____

_____

_____

_____

_____

_____

_____

_____

_____

Name _____   Specific Skill Performed _____
Date _____   Attempt Number _____
Instructor _____   PASS _____   FAIL _____

PERFORMANCE CHECKLIST 14.8   ADMINISTERING A CONTINUOUS-DRIP TUBE FEEDING

	S	U	COMMENTS
1. Checked physician's order, and type and rate of flow of feeding.			
2. Assessed for allergies, intolerances to formula ordered, client's weight, and electrolyte values.			
3. Explained procedure to client.			
4. Washed hands and used medical aseptic technique.			
5. Checked date of last change of administration set and tubing.			
6. Gathered appropriate equipment (i.e., formula, feeding bag, administration set).			
7. Closed clamp on administration set tubing.			
8. Connected administration set tubing to bottle of tube feeding solutions and hung bottle on IV pole.			
9. Connected administration set tubing to pump tubing and inserted into pump.			
10. Primed tubing correctly. Turned off pump.			
11. Raised head of bed 35° to 40° and placed drape under client's chin.			
12. Applied gloves.			
13. Checked tube placement correctly and checked for gastric residual.			
14. Attached pump tubing to nasogastric tube.			
15. Correctly set flow rate on pump and turned pump on.			
16. Observed flow of tube feeding.			
17. Removed and disposed of equipment appropriately.			
18. Removed gloves and washed hands.			
19. Documented procedure correctly.			

Name _____   Specific Skill Performed _____

Date _____   Attempt Number _____

Instructor _____   PASS _____   FAIL _____

PERFORMANCE CHECKLIST 14.9 IRRIGATING A NASOGASTRIC TUBE

	S	U	COMMENTS
1. Checked physician's order, and reason for tube. Assessed for contraindications to tube.			
2. Explained procedure to client.			
3. Assembled appropriate equipment (i.e., irrigant, irrigation tray, catheter-tipped syringe).			
4. Raised client to Fowler's position and placed drape across chest.			
5. Washed hands and applied gloves.			
6. Poured 30 to 200 ml. of irrigant into container.			
7. Provided privacy and placed bed at comfortable working height.			
8. Checked tubing for kinks and determined correct placement of tube in stomach.			
9. Filled syringe with correct solution for irrigation.			
10. Clamped tubing correctly and disconnected from connecting tube. Placed cap on end of connecting tube.			
11. Inserted tip of irrigating syringe into main lumen of tube and unclamped tube.			
12. Injected solution slowly and gently into tube.			
13. If resistance met, checked tubing for kinks, and had client turn. If resistance persisted, notified physician.			
14. After injecting solution into tube, withdrew fluid from tube.			
15. Instilled and withdrew fluid until fluid flowed freely.			
16. Reclamped tube to disconnect from irrigator. Reconnected to suction or feeding apparatus.			
17. Positioned client for comfort and safety.			
18. Observed tube for proper functioning.			

	S	U	COMMENTS
19. Cleaned or disposed of irrigation equipment appropriately.			
20. Removed gloves and washed hands.			
21. Documented irrigation time, amount and type of solution used, color, odor, consistency, and amount of drainage.			

Additional Comments:

_____

_____

_____

_____

_____

_____

_____

_____

_____

_____

_____

_____

_____

_____

_____

_____

_____

_____

_____

_____

Name _____   Specific Skill Performed _____
Date _____   Attempt Number _____
Instructor _____   PASS _____   FAIL _____

PERFORMANCE CHECKLIST 14.10 PROVIDING SITE CARE FOR A GASTROSTOMY TUBE, PERCUTANEOUS ENDOSCOPIC GASTROSTOMY TUBE, OR JEJUNOSTOMY TUBE

	S	U	COMMENTS
1. Assessed for presence of bowel sounds.			
2. Washed hands and applied gloves.			
3. Removed dressing if present and inspected skin around site.			
4. Inspected tube for migration in or out.			
5. Cleaned skin around tube correctly with peroxide and then antimicrobial soap.			
6. Rinsed and dried skin.			
7. Applied new dressing to tube insertion site.			
8. Documented procedure correctly.			

Additional Comments:

_____

_____

_____

_____

_____

_____

_____

_____

_____

_____

_____

Name _____   Specific Skill Performed _____
Date _____   Attempt Number _____
Instructor _____   PASS _____   FAIL _____

PERFORMANCE CHECKLIST 14.11 **ASSISTING WITH INSERTION OF A CENTRAL VENOUS LINE FOR ADMINISTRATION OF TOTAL PARENTERAL NUTRITION**

	S	U	COMMENTS
1. Explained procedure to client.			
2. Assessed client's nutritional and hydration status and vital signs.			
3. Assessed client's ability to hold his or her breath and tolerate Trendelenburg's position.			
4. Washed hands.			
5. Prepared 250 ml. bottle of D_5W properly and primed IV tubing.			
6. Prepared TPN infusion properly with infusion tubing primed and attached to pump and filter.			
7. Placed client in Trendelenburg position with rolled bath blanket under shoulders and head turned away from insertion site.			
8. Shaved insertion site if necessary.			
9. Put on mask and sterile gloves.			
10. Cleansed client's skin correctly with antiseptic solution.			
11. Removed gloves and discarded.			
12. Opened package of sterile gloves for physician.			
13. Opened package of sterile towels or sterile drape for physician.			
14. Opened 3 ml. syringe for physician.			
15. Swabbed rubber stopper for local anesthetic with alcohol, inverted bottle and held firmly while physician withdraws anesthetic.			
16. Opened packages containing catheter and 10 ml. syringe for physician.			
17. Explained procedure appropriately to client and asked client to perform Valsalva's maneuver.			
18. Once line in place, quickly connected IV line of D_5W to central venous line.			

	S	U	COMMENTS
19. Opened suture kit for physician.			
20. Applied sterile dressing to insertion site using correct procedure. Placed label with correct information on dressing.			
21. Prepared client for x-ray confirmation.			
22. After tube placement confirmed, disconnected D_5W and connected TPN correctly.			
23. Set the correct rate on infusion device for TPN.			
24. Evaluated client for signs of complications.			
25. Documented procedure correctly.			
26. Changed tubing according to hospital policy.			
27. Monitored infusion of TPN correctly.			

Additional Comments:

_____

_____

_____

_____

_____

_____

_____

_____

_____

_____

_____

_____

Name _____   Specific Skill Performed _____

Date _____   Attempt Number _____

Instructor _____   PASS _____   FAIL _____

PERFORMANCE CHECKLIST 14.12 PROVIDING SITE CARE FOR A CENTRAL VENOUS CATHETER

	S	U	COMMENTS
1. Gathered information regarding last dressing change and condition of insertion site.			
2. Explained procedure to client and helped client assume supine or semi-Fowler's position.			
3. Washed hands. Asked client to turn head away from insertion site.			
4. Opened sterile supplies and placed within easy reach.			
5. Removed dressing from insertion site and disposed of properly.			
6. Assessed condition of insertion site.			
7. Applied sterile gloves.			
8. Cleansed skin properly around insertion site and applied betadine ointment.			
9. Cleansed proximal tubing correctly.			
10. Ensured that all tubing connections are securely fastened.			
11. Removed gloves and applied new pair of sterile gloves.			
12. Applied sterile occlusive dressing correctly.			
13. Removed and discarded gloves.			
14. Labeled dressing correctly.			
15. Documented procedure correctly.			

Additional Comments:

_____

_____

_____

_____

_____

Name _____
Date _____
Instructor _____

Specific Skill Performed _____
Attempt Number _____
PASS _____   FAIL _____

PERFORMANCE CHECKLIST 15.1   **ADMINISTERING AN ENEMA**

	S	U	COMMENTS
1. Checked client chart for physician's order, rationale, diagnosis/ health problems, vital signs, and possible contraindications for enema administration.			
2. Collected appropriate equipment.			
3. Discussed procedure with client. Explained what to expect during and following the enema.			
4. Assessed client as needed.			
5. Warmed enema solution to 105° and checked temperature.			
6. Followed manufacturer's instructions to fill enema bag with solution. Primed the tubing, expelled all air, and lubricated the tip.			
7. Assisted client to bed and provided for privacy.			
8. Raised bed to comfortable working height.			
9. Put on gloves.			
10. Assisted client to left Sims position with waterproof pad under buttocks (knee-chest position for hypertonic solution). Draped client and exposed anus.			
11. Placed enema bag on IV pole at appropriate height.			
12. Separated the client's buttocks and inserted the enema tubing appropriately (2" for adult, 1/2 to 1" for child). Did not force tubing.			
13. Asked client to breathe deeply and slowly through the mouth.			
14. Released clamp and allowed solution to flow in slowly.			
15. If abdominal cramping occurred, stopped flow and instructed/ assisted client appropriately until cramping stopped.			
16. Administered appropriate amount of solution as ordered/according to client size and age.			
17. Clamped tubing and removed from client's rectum.			

	S	U	COMMENTS
18. Asked client to retain fluid for at least 5 minutes or as ordered/ indicated. Assisted client to retain fluid if needed (i.e., held buttocks together).			
19. Assisted client to bedpan or to bathroom.			
20. Stayed with client and observed for syncope, decreased heart rate and/or cardiac dysrhythmias.			
21. Instructed client/family not to flush toilet.			
22. Observed feces for amount, color, consistency, and odor.			
23. Properly cleansed client's rectal area.			
24. Assisted client to bed and positioned for comfort. Ensured that bed was in lowest position.			
25. Properly disposed/cleaned/stored equipment.			
26. Removed gloves and washed hands.			
27. Assessed client condition. Assessed enema results (if not done earlier).			
28. Documented the procedure including assessment data and client tolerance.			

Additional Comments:

_____

_____

_____

_____

_____

_____

_____

_____

_____

_____

Name _____
Date _____

Specific Skill Performed _____
Attempt Number _____

Instructor _____

PASS _____   FAIL _____

PERFORMANCE CHECKLIST 15.2   ADMINISTERING A PREPACKAGED ENEMA

	S	U	COMMENTS
1. Checked client's record for physician's order, rationale, diagnosis/ health problems, vital signs, and possible contraindications for enema administration.			
2. Obtained prepackaged enema as ordered and other needed equipment.			
3. Discussed procedure with client. Explained what to expect.			
4. Assessed client as needed.			
5. Provided privacy and assisted client to bed.			
6. Raised bed to comfortable working height.			
7. Put on gloves.			
8. Assisted client to left Sims position (knee-chest for hypertonic) with waterproof pad under buttocks. Draped client and exposed anus.			
9. Prepared enema for administration (i.e., removed tip, checked lubricant, expelled excess air, etc.).			
10. Separated client's buttocks and inserted enema tip appropriately (1 to 2"). Asked client to breathe deeply, slowly, and through his/her mouth during administration.			
11. Squeezed and rolled enema container toward client's rectum until all solution was administered.			
12. Removed container and asked client to retain solution for 5 to 10 minutes. Assisted client to retain fluid if needed (i.e., held buttocks together).			
13. Assisted client to bedpan or to bathroom.			
14. Stayed with client and observed for syncope, decreased heart rate and/or cardiac dysrhythmias.			
15. Instructed client/family not to flush toilet.			
16. Observed feces for amount, color, consistency, and odor.			
17. Properly cleansed client's rectal area.			

	S	U	COMMENTS
18. Assisted client to bed and positioned for comfort. Ensured that bed was in lowest position.			
19. Properly disposed/cleaned/stored equipment if appropriate.			
20. Removed gloves and washed hands.			
21. Assessed client's condition. Assessed enema results (if not done earlier).			
22. Documented the procedure including assessment data and client tolerance.			

Additional Comments:

_____

_____

_____

_____

_____

_____

_____

_____

_____

_____

_____

_____

_____

_____

_____

_____

_____

PERFORMANCE CHECKLIST 15.3   **REMOVING A FECAL IMPACTION**

	S	U	COMMENTS
1. Assessed client for presence of fecal impaction (i.e., last BM, liquid seepage of stool, abdominal distention) and determined need for removal.			
2. Assessed client's vital signs and health status.			
3. Checked client's record for physician's order to remove impaction. Checked agency policy manual.			
4. Gathered appropriate equipment.			
5. Discussed procedure with client. Explained what to expect.			
6. Provided privacy and assisted client to bed.			
7. Raised bed to comfortable working height.			
8. Put on gloves.			
9. Assisted client to left Sims position with waterproof pad under buttocks. Draped client and exposed anus.			
10. Placed bedpan beside client.			
11. Lubricated index finger and inserted it appropriately into anal canal.			
12. Felt for fecal mass. If present, used finger to break it up. Removed the small pieces and placed them in bedpan.			
13. Properly cleansed client's rectal area.			
14. Positioned client for comfort and returned bed to lowest position.			
15. Disposed of equipment appropriately.			
16. Removed gloves and washed hands.			
17. Assessed client's condition (i.e., vital signs, tolerance, etc.).			
18. Documented the procedure including assessment data and client tolerance of the procedure.			

Name _____ Specific Skill Performed _____

Date _____ Attempt Number _____

Instructor _____ PASS _____ FAIL _____

PERFORMANCE CHECKLIST 15.4   INSERTING A RECTAL TUBE

	S	U	COMMENTS
1. Assessed client's abdomen for distention and determined need.			
2. Checked client's chart for physician's order.			
3. Gathered appropriate equipment.			
4. Explained procedure to client.			
5. After assisting client to bed, raised the bed to comfortable working level and provided privacy.			
6. Positioned and draped client appropriately (i.e., left Sims with waterproof pad under buttocks and anus exposed.)			
7. Put on gloves.			
8. Lubricated tip of rectal tube.			
9. Separated client's buttocks and properly inserted rectal tube into rectum. Did not force insertion.			
10. Taped tube to one buttock. Placed open end of tube into plastic bag and closed it around tube (i.e., rubber band, etc.).			
11. Instructed client to remain on left side.			
12. Lowered bed and left tube in place for 20 to 30 minutes.			
13. After removal, properly cleaned client's rectal area.			
14. Removed gloves and washed hands.			
15. Assessed client for relief of distention.			
16. Positioned client for comfort and ensured that bed was in lowest position.			
17. Properly disposed of equipment. Re-washed hands.			
18. Documented the procedure including assessment data and client tolerance.			

Name _____   Specific Skill Performed _____
Date _____   Attempt Number _____
Instructor _____   PASS _____   FAIL _____

PERFORMANCE CHECKLIST 15.5   **ASSISTING WITH THE USE OF INCONTINENT BRIEFS**

	S	U	COMMENTS
1. Assessed client and checked chart to determine need.			
2. Gathered appropriate equipment/supplies.			
3. Discussed procedure with client, including rationale and client's feelings about procedure (if initiating treatment).			
4. Assisted client to bed. Raised bed to comfortable working height and provided privacy.			
5. Put on gloves and placed waterproof pad under client's buttocks/hips.			
6. If present, removed soiled briefs and discarded them appropriately.			
7. Cleaned and dried client's perineum and surrounding skin (i.e., area covered by briefs).			
8. Assessed client's skin for evidence of irritation/breakdown.			
9. Provided protection to skin as ordered/per protocol (i.e., ointment, medication, etc.).			
10. Removed waterproof pad if soiled.			
11. Properly placed open, clean briefs under client's hips/buttocks and fastened them appropriately at the client's waist (i.e., diapering action).			
12. Disposed of gloves (if not already done).			
13. Positioned client for comfort and ensured that bed was in lowest position.			
14. Washed hands.			
15. Documented the procedure including assessment data and client tolerance.			

Additional Comments:

_____

_____

_____

Name _____   Specific Skill Performed _____
Date _____   Attempt Number _____
Instructor _____   PASS _____   FAIL _____

PERFORMANCE CHECKLIST 15.6   DIAPERING AN INFANT

	S	U	COMMENTS
1. Assessed infant and determined need.			
2. Gathered equipment.			
3. Washed hands and put on gloves.			
4. Placed child on firm surface at comfortable working height (i.e., bed or changing table). Kept hands on child and did not turn away at any time.			
5. Removed soiled diaper, assessed contents and discarded appropriately according to agency protocol.			
6. Cleansed infant's skin appropriately.			
7. Assessed infant's skin in diaper area (i.e., for redness, rash, breakdown, etc.).			
8. Applied protective barrier to skin if needed/appropriate.			
9. Applied new diaper and fastened securely.			
10. Removed gloves and discarded appropriately.			
11. Ensured client safety.			
12. Washed hands.			
13. Documented procedure and assessment data.			

Additional Comments:

_____

_____

_____

_____

_____

_____

_____

Name _____   Specific Skill Performed _____
Date _____   Attempt Number _____
Instructor _____   PASS _____   FAIL _____

PERFORMANCE CHECKLIST 15.7   CARING FOR A STOMA

	S	U	COMMENTS
1. Checked chart/assessed client to determine type of ostomy.			
2. Collected appropriate supplies.			
3. Discussed procedure with client/family. Assessed client/family readiness to learn about ostomy care.			
4. Assisted client to bed, provided privacy, and raised bed to comfortable working height.			
5. Assisted client to supine or sitting position with stoma exposed and bed/clothes protected.			
6. Put on gloves.			
7. Informed/explained each step to client.			
8. Massaged client's proximal intestine toward stoma.			
9. Emptied ostomy appliance (collection bag) into bedpan. Assessed fecal drainage.			
10. Loosened skin barrier appropriately.			
11. Supported client's skin while properly removing barrier and bag (i.e., gently, diagonally away from hands, etc.).			
12. Covered stoma after bag removed (i.e., toilet paper, etc.).			
13. Discarded used appliance according to agency protocol (i.e., sealed in plastic bag, etc.).			
14. Properly cleaned the stoma (clear water) and surrounding skin (soap and water). Rinsed area and patted it dry. Did not rub skin or stoma.			
15. Assessed the stoma and the surrounding skin.			
16. Correctly measured the stoma and prepared the skin barrier to fit (i.e., cut out hole the size of stoma).			
17. Correctly prepared the appliance to fit over stoma (i.e., cut hole 1/8" to 1/4" larger than stoma) and attached to skin barrier. Smoothed barrier to remove all air bubbles.			

	S	U	COMMENTS
18. Used skin paste as needed to fill irregularities in stoma border (before placing barrier/appliance over stoma).			
19. Removed the paper from the adhesive side of the skin barrier and correctly applied it around stoma (i.e., bag in dependent position). Smoothed skin barrier all around stoma.			
20. Added odor controller to bag if needed.			
21. Properly closed/fastened end of bag with clamp.			
22. Used waterproof 1" tape to make a "picture frame" around the outer edges of the appliance,.			
23. Assessed appliance for fit and leakage.			
24. Positioned client for comfort and lowered bed.			
25. Disposed of soiled equipment.			
26. Removed gloves and washed hands.			
27. Documented the procedure including assessment data, client response and any teaching-learning activities.			

Additional Comments:

_____

_____

_____

_____

_____

_____

_____

_____

_____

_____

_____

Name _____   Specific Skill Performed _____
Date _____   Attempt Number _____
Instructor _____   PASS _____   FAIL _____

PERFORMANCE CHECKLIST 15.8 CARING FOR A CONTINENT ILEOSTOMY

	S	U	COMMENTS
1. Assessed client for readiness to learn and to determine need. Discussed procedure with client.			
2. Gathered equipment.			
3. Provided privacy and assisted client to proper position for ileostomy catheterization (i.e., toilet, bedside commode, bedpan at bedside) with ileostomy exposed.			
4. Put on gloves.			
5. Informed/explained each step to client.			
6. Removed ileostomy dressing and disposed of properly.			
7. Lubricated 3" of the catheter.			
8. Placed distal end of catheter into receptacle (i.e., toilet or bedpan).			
9. Properly inserted catheter into ileostomy (i.e., downward 2") until resistance is felt.			
10. Instructed client to take a deep breath and inserted the catheter through the outlet valve into the pouch reservoir.			
11. Drained all contents from pouch.			
12. Irrigated catheter and pouch with 30 to 50 ml. of normal saline in 50 ml. syringe if needed.			
13. Cleaned stoma and surrounding skin with soap and water. Rinsed area well and patted it dry. Did not rub skin or stoma.			
14. Placed clean 4 x 4 gauze over stoma and secured it with tape.			
15. Assisted client to position of comfort and ensured that bed was lowered.			
16. Cleaned and disposed of equipment appropriately.			
17. Removed gloves and washed hands.			
18. Documented the procedure including assessment data, client response, and any teaching-learning activities.			

Name _____   Specific Skill Performed _____
Date _____   Attempt Number _____
Instructor _____   PASS _____   FAIL _____

PERFORMANCE CHECKLIST 15.9   **PERFORMING A COLOSTOMY IRRIGATION**

	S	U	COMMENTS
1. Checked client's chart for physician's order to begin irrigations and to determine type of ostomy.			
2. Discussed procedure with client/family. Determined when irrigation to be done (i.e., best time of day for client). Assessed client readiness to learn procedure.			
3. Gathered equipment.			
4. Provided privacy and assisted client to proper position (i.e., toilet, bedside commode, bedpan at bedside) with ostomy area exposed.			
5. Adjusted water temperature (104°) and filled irrigation bag with water (500 to 1000 ml.). Ensured that temperature was correct.			
6. Hung irrigation bag at client's shoulder level, purged the tubing of air and closed the clamp.			
7. Put on gloves.			
8. Emptied appliance into receptacle (i.e., toilet, bedside commode, or bedpan) and assessed the fecal material.			
9. Loosened the skin barrier appropriately.			
10. Supported client's skin while properly removing barrier and bag (i.e., gently, diagonally away from hands, etc.).			
11. Discarded used appliance according to agency policy.			
12. Assessed stoma and surrounding skin.			
13. Placed belt around client. Attached irrigation sleeve and placed distal end into receptacle.			
14. Lubricated the cone and inserted it through the top opening of the irrigation sleeve into the stoma. Did not force entry.			
15. Released the clamp on the irrigation tubing and let water flow slowly into intestines (i.e., over 15 minutes). If abdominal cramping occurred, closed clamp and let client rest before resuming flow.			

	S	U	COMMENTS
16. When irrigation completed, removed cone and folded down/ secured top of sleeve with clip. Ensured that distal end of sleeve remained in receptacle.			
17. Instructed client to remain in position for 15 minutes (with emergency call within reach).			
18. After 15 minutes, clamped bottom of sleeve and left it in place for 1 hour. Assisted client to bed if needed or allowed client to ambulate with sleeve in place.			
19. At appropriate time, removed irrigation sleeve and emptied, cleaned, and stored it properly.			
20. Cleaned stoma and skin around it with soap and water. Rinsed well and patted it dry. Did not rub area.			
21. Properly placed a clean appliance over stoma.			
22. Removed gloves and washed hands.			
23. Documented the procedure including assessment data, client response, and any teaching-learning activities.			

Additional Comments:

_____

_____

_____

_____

_____

_____

_____

_____

_____

_____

_____

Name _____   Specific Skill Performed _____
Date _____   Attempt Number _____
Instructor _____   PASS _____   FAIL _____

PERFORMANCE CHECKLIST 16.1   **MEASURING URINARY OUTPUT**

	S	U	COMMENTS
1. Assessed client's ability to learn.			
2. Gathered appropriate materials (i.e., graduated container or urinal, gloves, intake and output sheet).			
3. Put on gloves.			
4. Collected client's urine. Poured urine into graduated container from urinal or catheter drainage bag if necessary.			
5. Measured urine in graduated container correctly.			
6. Assessed color, odor, and clarity or urine.			
7. Emptied urine into toilet.			
8. Rinsed measuring device and returned to storage.			
9. Removed gloves and washed hands.			
10. Recorded amount of urine on output side of intake and output sheet. Recorded assessment of urine on progress notes.			

Additional Comments:

_____

_____

_____

_____

_____

_____

_____

_____

_____

_____

Name _____   Specific Skill Performed _____

Date _____   Attempt Number _____

Instructor _____   PASS _____   FAIL _____

PERFORMANCE CHECKLIST 16.2   **ASSISTING THE CLIENT WITH A BEDPAN OR FRACTURE PAN**

	S	U	COMMENTS
1. Washed hands.			
2. Assessed client's mobility and ability to assist with using bedpan. Obtained assistance if necessary.			
3. Explained procedure to client.			
4. Gathered appropriate materials, (i.e., bedpan, toilet tissue, washcloth and towel).			
5. Raised bed to comfortable working height. Raised distal side rail and lowered proximal side rail.			
6. Provided for client privacy.			
7. Positioned client's bed flat with client on back.			
8. Instructed client to flex knees and push with feet to raise buttocks.			
9. Slid bedpan under client's buttocks in proper position.			
10. If client unable to assist, rolled client toward far side of bed.			
11. Placed bedpan against client's buttocks. Pushed downward on bedpan while rolling client onto back on bedpan.			
12. Checked to be sure bedpan is positioned in center and covered client with top linen.			
13. If allowed, raised head of bed to sitting position.			
14. Raised side rail and put call light in reach. Instructed client not to put toilet paper in bedpan if output is to be measured or specimen collected.			
15. To remove bedpan, put on gloves and positioned bed flat.			
16. Asked client to lift buttocks or rolled client to far side while holding bedpan securely.			
17. Slid bedpan out and helped client cleanse perineal area, if necessary.			
18. Replaced client's gown and top linens.			

	S	U	COMMENTS
19. Offered client clean, wet washcloth and towel to cleanse hands.			
20. Emptied bedpan into toilet after measuring urine. Cleansed bedpan.			
21. Removed gloves and washed hands.			
22. Returned clean, dry bedpan to storage.			
23. Recorded amount, color, and consistency of urine or feces.			

Additional Comments:

_____

_____

_____

_____

_____

_____

_____

_____

_____

_____

_____

_____

_____

_____

_____

_____

_____

_____

Name _____   Specific Skill Performed _____

Date _____   Attempt Number _____

Instructor _____   PASS _____   FAIL _____

PERFORMANCE CHECKLIST 16.3   ASSISTING THE MALE CLIENT WITH A URINAL

	S	U	COMMENTS
1. Checked for restriction in client's movement.			
2. Provided for client privacy.			
3. Washed hands and put on gloves.			
4. If client confined to bed, assisted to appropriate position with urinal between legs and client's penis in urinal.			
5. If client able to stand, helped him assume a standing position and handed urinal to him.			
6. Placed call light within client's reach.			
7. After voiding completed, removed urinal, emptied it, measured urine and rinsed out urinal.			
8. Helped client clean himself. Offered clean washcloth for handwashing.			
9. Removed gloves and washed hands.			
10. Recorded color, amount and odor of urine.			

Additional Comments:

_____

_____

_____

_____

_____

_____

_____

_____

Name _____   Specific Skill Performed _____
Date _____   Attempt Number _____
Instructor _____   PASS _____   FAIL _____

PERFORMANCE CHECKLIST 16.4   **INSERTING AN INDWELLING CATHETER**

	S	U	COMMENTS
1. Checked physician's order and need for catheterization.			
2. Assessed client's ability to follow directions and cooperate. Obtained assistance if necessary.			
3. Washed hands.			
4. Gathered necessary equipment (i.e., catheter insertion kit, washcloth, and towel, proper lighting, correct catheter).			
5. Explained procedure to client and provided for privacy.			
6. Raised bed to comfortable working height and lowered proximal side rail.			
7. Placed client in appropriate position and draped. Placed waterproof pad under client's buttocks.			
8. Washed, rinsed, and dried genital area.			
9. Positioned light source to provide maximum visibility.			
10. Using sterile technique, opened sterile prepackaged catheter insertion kit at the appropriate site for the gender and level of cooperation of the client.			
11. Removed sterile pad, opened it at the corners without contaminating it and placed it in the appropriate position.			
12. Removed sterile gloves from package and applied correctly.			
13. Removed fenestrated drape and placed it so that only the genitals are exposed.			
14. Opened disinfectant solution and poured over cotton balls.			
15. Attached prefilled syringe to balloon port. Tested balloon then kept syringe in place at balloon port.			
16. Opened lubricant and lubricated tip of catheter correctly.			
17. For female client, spread the labia with nondominant hand and did not allow labia to close during procedure. For male client, used nondominant hand to position penis perpendicular to body.			

	S	U	COMMENTS
18. Grasping forceps in dominant hand, picked up cottonball containing disinfectant. Cleansed meatus correctly.			
19. Visualized the urinary meatus, picked up catheter with sterile hand and inserted into meatus gently and without contaminating it.			
20. Inserted catheter 2 to 3 inches for adult females and to the bifurcation for adult males. Made sure urine is flowing out through catheter.			
21. Injected sterile water into balloon port according to the amount specified.			
22. Gently tugged on catheter to be sure balloon was inflated. Disconnected syringe.			
23. Attached catheter to drainage bag, if necessary. Attached drainage bag to frame of bed below level of client's bladder.			
24. Returned foreskin to correct position on uncircumcised males.			
25. Removed gloves and washed hands.			
26. Coiled extra tubing on bed to avoid kinks or dependent loops.			
27. Taped catheter tubing correctly to protect from pulling.			
28. Cleansed client's perineum, removed drapes, and placed client in position of comfort and safety.			
29. Returned bed to lowest position and replaced bed covers.			
30. Removed and properly disposed of contaminated equipment.			
31. Documented procedure, client's response, and assessment of urine.			

Additional Comments:

_____

_____

_____

_____

_____

_____

_____

Name _____   Specific Skill Performed _____
Date _____   Attempt Number _____
Instructor _____   PASS _____   FAIL _____

PERFORMANCE CHECKLIST 16.5   PROVIDING HYGIENIC CARE FOR A CLIENT WITH AN INDWELLING CATHETER

	S	U	COMMENTS
1. Explained procedure to client.			
2. Assessed for signs of urinary tract infection or need for catheter change.			
3. Provided for client privacy.			
4. Washed hands and put on gloves.			
5. Positioned client correctly.			
6. Draped client and slid waterproof pad in place.			
7. Used warm soapy water to cleanse urinary meatus and catheter.			
8. Rinsed and dried perineum. Assessed for signs of irritation, trauma or secretions.			
9. Removed waterproof pad and replaced gown and top linens.			
10. Removed gloves and washed hands.			
11. Checked tubing for proper positioning and made sure urine was free-flowing.			
12. Documented procedure, client's response, and assessment of catheter and urine.			

Additional Comments:

_____

_____

_____

_____

_____

_____

_____

_____

Name _____   Specific Skill Performed _____
Date _____   Attempt Number _____
Instructor _____   PASS _____   FAIL _____

PERFORMANCE CHECKLIST 16.6   **REMOVING AN INDWELLING CATHETER**

	S	U	COMMENTS
1. Checked physician's order and assessed length of time catheter has been in place.			
2. Explained procedure to client.			
3. Gathered appropriate equipment (i.e., syringe, towel).			
4. Washed hands and applied gloves.			
5. Provided for privacy and draped client. Positioned client to allow for good visualization of the perineum.			
6. Slid waterproof pad under meatus.			
7. Inserted syringe or needle into balloon sleeve valve and withdrew all fluid from catheter balloon.			
8. Asked client to take deep breath and gently removed catheter.			
9. Inspected balloon to be sure it is intact.			
10. Assessed meatus for signs of infection or edema. Cleaned and dried perineum.			
11. Removed waterproof pad and positioned client for comfort and safety.			
12. Instructed client to inform you when needing to void.			
13. Measured urine in drainage bag. Disposed of equipment properly.			
14. Removed gloves and washed hands.			
15. When client voided, noted amount and color of urine, and the presence of any sediment.			
16. Documented removal of catheter, condition of meatus, and client response to procedure.			

Additional Comments:

_____

_____

_____

Name _____   Specific Skill Performed _____
Date _____   Attempt Number _____
Instructor _____   PASS _____   FAIL _____

PERFORMANCE CHECKLIST 16.7   **APPLYING A CONDOM CATHETER**

	S	U	COMMENTS
1. Explained procedure to client.			
2. Gathered appropriate equipment (i.e., condom catheter, drainage bag).			
3. Washed hands and applied gloves.			
4. Provided for client privacy and raised bed to comfortable working height. Placed client in supine position.			
5. Assessed penis for signs of irritation or skin breakdown.			
6. Washed penis and perineum with soap and water and dried well.			
7. Shaved perineum if pubic hair excessive.			
8. Applied skin prep wipe to shaft of penis.			
9. Correctly applied adhesive strip to base of penis in a spiral fashion.			
10. Unrolled condom sheath smoothly over penis, leaving a 0.5-inch to 1-inch gap between distal end of penis and connecting tube. Gently pressed to adhesive strip.			
11. Attached condom to drainage bag and drainage bag to bed frame or to leg as appropriate. Secured excess tubing.			
12. Positioned client for comfort and safety.			
13. Disposed of used equipment appropriately.			
14. Removed gloves and washed hands.			
15. Assessed urinary output.			
16. Documented procedure.			

Additional Comments:

_____

_____

_____

_____

Name _____

Date _____

Instructor _____

Specific Skill Performed _____

Attempt Number _____

PASS _____   FAIL _____

PERFORMANCE CHECKLIST 16.8   **PERFORMING CONTINUOUS BLADDER IRRIGATION**

	S	U	COMMENTS
1. Checked physician's order for irrigation and medical diagnosis of client.			
2. Washed hands.			
3. Provided for client privacy.			
4. Connected tubing to irrigation fluid bag using sterile technique.			
5. Allowed fluid to flow through tubing until air removed. Closed clamp. Squeezed drip chamber 1/3 to 1/2 full.			
6. Hung irrigation bag on IV pole 3 feet above bladder.			
7. Connected irrigation tubing to inflow port of catheter using sterile technique.			
8. Attached urinary drainage bag to outflow port, if necessary.			
9. Opened irrigation clamp and adjusted rate as ordered.			
10. After 15 minutes, assessed client and drainage.			
11. Calculated urinary output correctly.			
12. Documented procedure correctly.			

Additional Comments:

_____

_____

_____

_____

_____

_____

_____

_____

_____

PERFORMANCE CHECKLIST 16.9   **CARING FOR THE CLIENT WITH A URINARY DIVERSION**

	S	U	COMMENTS
1. Assessed client's knowledge level and readiness to learn.			
2. Provided for client privacy.			
3. Raised bed to comfortable working height.			
4. Placed client in supine or sitting position. Protected client and bed with waterproof pad.			
5. Washed hands and applied gloves.			
6. Explained procedure to client.			
7. Emptied appliance and assessed urine.			
8. Loosened skin barrier using alcohol soaked pad.			
9. Gently pulled barrier and bag away from client while supporting skin.			
10. Placed used appliance in plastic bag and discarded it appropriately.			
11. Covered opening of stoma with gauze pad, while washing skin around stoma with mild soap and water.			
12. Rinsed and patted area dry. Assessed stoma and surrounding skin.			
13. Cut proper size hole in skin barrier.			
14. Placed appliance over skin barrier correctly, smoothing the adhesive to remove air bubbles.			
15. Filled in irregular borders of stoma with karaya paste and removed gauze pad from stoma.			
16. Applied appliance and skin barrier unit around stoma correctly attaching dependent edge first.			
17. Smoothed down adhesive around stoma and closed outlet port at bottom of appliance.			
18. Secured with waterproof tape around outer edges.			

	S	U	COMMENTS
19. Positioned client for comfort and safety.			
20. Disposed of equipment properly.			
21. Removed gloves and washed hands.			
22. Checked to determine proper adherence of appliance and that it was not leaking.			
23. Answered client's questions regarding procedure.			
24. Documented procedure and condition of skin and stoma.			

Additional Comments:

_____

_____

_____

_____

_____

_____

_____

_____

_____

_____

_____

_____

_____

_____

_____

_____

_____

Name _____   Specific Skill Performed _____
Date _____   Attempt Number _____
Instructor _____   PASS _____   FAIL _____

PERFORMANCE CHECKLIST 17.1   **ASSESSING OXYGENATION STATUS WITH ARTERIAL BLOOD GASES**

	S	U	COMMENTS
1. Assessed client condition and determined need. Checked chart for physician's order/standing order/agency protocol re: ABGs.			
2. Checked client's medication record re: anticoagulant therapy. Determined if client had an arterial line in place.			
3. Gathered appropriate equipment and explained procedure to client/family.			
4. Checked client's vital signs and temperature.			
5. Assessed appropriate arterial sites for availability, etc. (preferred site in adult: radial).			
6. Checked for alternative circulation to hand by properly performing Allen's test (i.e., occluded both radial and ulnar arteries, released ulnar and observed for return of blood flow to hand). Checked other hand if needed.			
7. Assessed other conditions that may effect ABG results (i.e., changes in O_2 settings, recent suctioning, client's activities and emotions).			
8. Placed supplies for convenient use and prepared equipment (i.e., heparinized syringe, cup with ice, etc.).			
9. Assisted client to position of comfort and raised bed to comfortable working height with side rail down if needed.			
Performing Arterial Puncture and Specimen Collection			
10. Provided support for client as needed during specimen withdrawal.			
11. Washed hands and put on gloves.			
12. Placed waterproof pad under client's hand and hyperextended it.			
13. Cleaned puncture site according to agency policy.			
14. Located radial artery. Placed index finger (non-dominant hand) on one side of artery and middle finger along other side.			
15. Asked client to remain very still during puncture.			

	S	U	COMMENTS
16. Used appropriate technique to insert needle and observed for flashback. Did not pull back on plunger.			
17. If unsuccessful, used appropriate technique to redirect needle for puncture. Did not withdraw needle.			
18. Withdrew 3 to 5 ml. blood.			
19. Removed needle and applied pressure to site for 5 minutes (10 minutes if client on anticoagulant therapy) and then placed dressing over site if needed.			
20. Expelled air bubbles from syringe (while maintaining pressure on site), stuck needle into rubber stopper, rotated syringe gently and placed in cup of ice.			
21. Correctly labeled and prepared specimen for transport to lab for analysis (i.e., iced specimen in biohazard bag, etc.).			
22. Removed gloves and washed hands.			
23. Lowered bed and raised side rail if needed.			
24. Completed requisition including assessment data and pertinent information and sent/took specimen to lab immediately.			
25. Inspected puncture site periodically.			
26. Evaluated the ABG results when available.			
27. Documented the procedure including assessment data, client response and results of analysis.			
28. Informed appropriate persons of results if indicated.			

Additional Comments:

_____

_____

_____

_____

_____

_____

_____

_____

Name _____   Specific Skill Performed _____
Date _____   Attempt Number _____
Instructor _____   PASS _____   FAIL _____

PERFORMANCE CHECKLIST 17.2   **ASSESSING OXYGENATION STATUS WITH PULSE OXIMETRY**

	S	U	COMMENTS
1. Assessed client condition, including hemoglobin level, and followed physician order/agency policy regarding use of pulse oximetry.			
2. Gathered equipment.			
3. Discussed procedure with client/family. Explained what to expect and instructed client to avoid moving extremity with sensor on it.			
4. Selected appropriate sensor.			
5. Selected appropriate site with adequate circulation and good proximal pulse.			
6. Properly prepared site.			
7. Correctly applied sensor.			
8. Connected sensor to oximeter and turned on machine. Checked for appropriate tone and waveform and set the alarms according to manufacturer's directions.			
9. Protected the sensor from bright light.			
10. Changed the sensor site according to agency protocol (i.e., spring sensor at q 2 hrs., adhesive sensor at q 4 hrs.).			
11. Notified the physician of abnormal results.			
12. Documented the procedure including assessment data, Hgb level, results of the O_2 saturation measurements, type of sensor used and skin conditions at sensor site.			

Additional Comments:

_____

_____

_____

_____

_____

Name _____
Date _____

Specific Skill Performed _____
Attempt Number _____

Instructor _____

PASS _____   FAIL _____

PERFORMANCE CHECKLIST 17.3   **ADMINISTERING OXYGEN BY NASAL CANNULA, MASK, NASAL CATHETER, AND CROUPETTE, MIST TENT, OR OXYGEN TENT**

	S	U	COMMENTS
1. Assessed client condition (i.e., respiratory status, vital signs, etc.). Determined need.			
2. Checked client's chart for physician's order, diagnosis and relevant health problems (i.e., COPD).			
3. Assessed pertinent lab results (i.e., ABGs, Hgb, etc.).			
4. Gathered appropriate equipment.			
5. Explained procedure and purpose of oxygen therapy to client/family including necessary precautions (i.e., "No Smoking").			
6. Inserted flowmeter into oxygen outlet (or set up oxygen tank).			
7. Properly connected humidification bottle to flowmeter. Filled reservoir with distilled water if not pre-filled.			
8. Connected oxygen tubing and delivery device to outlet port on humidifier bottle.			
9. Adjusted flowmeter to deliver oxygen at 2 LPM and checked to see if oxygen was flowing through system.			
10. Positioned oxygen delivery device on client.			
Administering Oxygen with a Nasal Cannula			
11. Placed nasal prongs just inside client's nares and secured cannula according to manufacturer's directions (i.e., looped around ears and adjusted under chin.			
12. Instructed client to breathe through nose.			
Administering Oxygen with a Mask			
13. Placed appropriate mask over client's nose and mouth. Secured it with elastic strap around back of head.			

	S	U	COMMENTS
Administering Oxygen with a Nasal Catheter			
14. Correctly measured/marked amount of catheter to be inserted into client's nostril.			
15. Put on gloves.			
16. Appropriately lubricated catheter.			
17. Assessed patency of nares and gently placed catheter into the one determined to be most open.			
18. Properly inserted catheter for pre-determined length and temporarily secured it with tape to client's nose.			
19. Checked placement of catheter and adjusted it as needed (i.e., used penlight/tongue blade to examine back of client's throat).			
20. Securely fastened nasal catheter to client's nose.			
21. Removed gloves and discarded them.			
22. Changed catheter every 8 hours and positioned it in different place (i.e., used other nostril if possible).			
All Administration Modes			
23. Adjusted flowmeter to rate as ordered by physician.			
24. Observed the effects of oxygen on client (i.e., assessed ABGs, pulse oximetry, respiratory rate/pattern and changes in level of consciousness).			
25. Washed hands.			
26. Posted "No Smoking" sign.			
27. Documented the procedure, including assessment data and client response.			
28. Periodically checked on equipment to ensure proper operation (i.e., oxygen flow rate settings, water in reservoir, kinks in tubing, etc.).			

	S	U	COMMENTS
Administering Oxygen with a Croupette, Mist Tent or Oxygen Tent			
29. Assessed client condition, including respiratory status, ABGs, vital signs, ability to clear airway of secretion, and anxiety level for both client and family.			
30. Checked client's chart for physician's orders, diagnosis, and other relevant information.			
31. Gathered equipment and took to bedside.			
32. Explained procedure, equipment and purpose of oxygen therapy to client and family including necessary precautions.			
33. Washed hands. Put on gloves if needed.			
34. Placed nebulizer or humidifier at bedside, connected canopy nd covered bed/crib. Connected unit securely to oxygen source.			
35. Turned on refrigeration unit (or stocked reservoir with ice).			
36. Followed manufacturer's directions to fill nebulizer or humidifier and set flowmeter for oxygen delivery.			
37. Dressed child appropriately before placing inside tent or canopy (i.e., extra clothes if air cooled by refrigerator/ice).			
38. Placed child in high-Fowler's or semi-Fowler's position inside tent with a non-hazardous, developmentally appropriate toy. Placed tissues and disposal bag in tent with older child.			
39. Tucked top and sides of canopy/tent under mattress and placed top sheet over front section of tent.			
40. Placed "No Smoking"/"Oxygen in Use" signs on door and over bed.			
41. Encouraged family participation in care. Planned nursing care so that tent would be opened as infrequently as possible. Flushed tent with oxygen when reclosing it after extended open period and then resumed prescribed settings.			
42. Frequently evaluated client's needs and condition. Frequently checked the equipment.			
43. Documented the procedures including assessment data and client response.			

Name _____   Specific Skill Performed _____

Date _____   Attempt Number _____

Instructor _____   PASS _____   FAIL _____

PERFORMANCE CHECKLIST 17.4   **ORAL AND NASAL CARE FOR A CLIENT WHO IS RECEIVING OXYGEN**

	S	U	COMMENTS
1. Assessed client condition (i.e., integrity of mucous membrane) and determined need.			
2. Gathered equipment.			
3. Explained procedure and purpose to client.			
4. Put on gloves.			
5. Provided alternative source of oxygen to client with mask if needed (i.e., nasal cannula) while giving oral care.			
6. Assisted with oral care as needed.			
7. Appropriately cleaned client's nostrils and allowed client to blow nose gently. Gently lubricated client's lips and nares.			
8. Reapplied the oxygen delivery device in slightly different position if possible.			
9. Padded area under head strap above ears and between client's nose and cannula if needed.			
10. Removed gloves. Washed hands.			
11. Ensured that oxygen settings were correctly set and checked client comfort.			
12. Documented the procedure including assessment data and client response.			

Additional Comments:

_____

_____

_____

_____

_____

_____

Name _____   Specific Skill Performed _____
Date _____   Attempt Number _____
Instructor _____   PASS _____   FAIL _____

PERFORMANCE CHECKLIST 17.5   **ASSISTING A CLIENT WITH DEEP BREATHING, COUGHING, AND BREATHING TECHNIQUES**

	S	U	COMMENTS
Teaching Deep Breathing			
1. Explained procedure and importance to client.			
2. Assisted client to sitting position (i.e., on side of bed or in high-Fowler's position).			
3. Had client inhale slowly as deeply as possible. Assessed client's chest excursion.			
4. Had client exhale slowly.			
5. Repeated steps 3 and 4 for 10 to 20 times. Observed client for dizziness, shortness of breath, and other respiratory problems.			
Helping the Client to Cough			
6. Explained procedure and its importance.			
7. Assisted client to sitting position (i.e., side of bed or in high-Fowler's position).			
8. Put on protective gear if appropriate (i.e., mask, etc.).			
9. Appropriately assisted client to cough forcefully and effectively (i.e., splinted client's chest/abdomen and had client lean forward, hold breath, contract abdominal muscles and cough/expectorate into tissue/basin).			
10. Assessed client's lungs by auscultation (i.e., for removal of secretions).			
11. Disposed of tissues. Cleaned basin.			
12. Provided mouth care if needed and assisted client to position of comfort.			
13. Removed protective gear and washed hands.			
14. Encouraged client to increase fluid intake (if not contraindicated).			

	S	U	COMMENTS
Teaching Pursed-Lip Breathing			
15. Explained purpose for pursed-lip breathing.			
16. Had client inhale through nose and then purse lips (i.e., as if to kiss someone).			
17. Instructed client to exhale slowly through pursed lips.			
Teaching Diaphragmatic Breathing			
18. Assisted client to position of comfort.			
19. Had client place hands correctly (i.e., upper abdomen and upper chest) to monitor diaphragmatic movement.			
20. Had client consciously pull upward with abdominal muscles during exhalation.			
21. Had client consciously pull diaphragm down during inhalation.			
22. Observe client for untoward effects (i.e., dizziness, shortness of breath, etc.).			
All Breathing Techniques			
23. Documented procedure/activity in client's records, including assessment data, client response and any teaching-learning activities.			

Additional Comments:

_____

_____

_____

_____

_____

_____

_____

_____

Name _____

Date _____

Instructor _____

Specific Skill Performed _____

Attempt Number _____

PASS _____   FAIL _____

PERFORMANCE CHECKLIST 17.6   **ASSISTING A CLIENT WITH AN INCENTIVE SPIROMETER**

	S	U	COMMENTS
1. Reviewed client's chart for diagnosis, orders, history of respiratory problems, laboratory results (i.e., ABGs), and pre-operative respiratory status (i.e., inspiratory volume).			
2. Assessed client condition (i.e., respiratory status, comfort level) and medicated client for pain if necessary.			
3. Gathered equipment.			
4. Explained procedure and purpose to client (i.e., reinforced pre-op teaching, etc.).			
5. Assisted client to position of comfort (i.e., semi- or high-Fowler's position in bed or chair). Raised bed to comfortable working height if client remained in bed.			
6. Had client exhale and then cover mouthpiece completely with lips to form an adequate seal.			
7. Instructed client to inhale slowly and deeply through nose while maintaining the seal over the mouthpiece. Also instructed client to watch the ball or gauge rise to the desired/preset point during inhalation.			
8. At the end of inhalation, had client hold breath for 3 seconds before exhalation.			
9. Had client take 2 to 4 normal breaths between attempts and repeat the procedure 10 to 20 times.			
10. Instructed client to report any dizziness, shortness of breath, etc., and that incentive spirometry should be done every hour while awake.			
11. Assisted client to position of comfort and ensured that bed was in low position.			
12. Assessed the client's respiratory status, including sputum production.			
13. Removed/cleaned mouthpiece and stored it appropriately.			
14. Documented the procedure, including assessment data, client response and any teaching-learning activities.			

Name _____   Specific Skill Performed _____
Date _____   Attempt Number _____
Instructor _____   PASS _____   FAIL _____

PERFORMANCE CHECKLIST 17.7   **USING A HUMIDIFIER**

		S	U	COMMENTS
1.	Checked client's chart for physician's order, diagnosis, and rationale for the use of a humidifier.			
2.	Collected equipment. Checked humidifier to see if it was in good operating condition (i.e., checked cord, plug, ground wire, moving parts, etc.).			
3.	Explained to the client the purpose for using a humidifier.			
4.	Followed manufacturer's direction to assemble/set up the humidifier (i.e., filled with distilled water, placed on table near client, plugged into grounded outlet, etc.).			
5.	Ensured that humidifier location would not be a safety hazard. Protected table top from excess moisture (i.e., put towel under humidifier).			
6.	Turned on humidifier and watched for mist to begin. Adjusted mist level according to manufacturer's directions.			
7.	Instructed client to remain in room in order to get beneficial effects of humidifier.			
8.	Washed hands.			
9.	Documented procedure.			
10.	Periodically checked the humidifier's water level and refilled if needed.			
11.	Cleaned humidifier every 24 hours according to manufacturer's directions.			

Additional Comments:

_____

_____

_____

_____

_____

_____

Name _____   Specific Skill Performed _____

Date _____   Attempt Number _____

Instructor _____   PASS _____   FAIL _____

PERFORMANCE CHECKLIST 17.8   PROVIDING CHEST PHYSIOTHERAPY

	S	U	COMMENTS
1. Assessed client condition (i.e., heart and breath sounds, respiratory pattern, and secretions) and comfort level.			
2. Checked client's record for physician's order/rationale. Reviewed history for health conditions, problems, and possible contraindications for chest P-T (i.e., ICP, pulmonary edema, abdominal complications, etc.).			
3. Determined which lung segments required treatment.			
4. Gathered appropriate equipment.			
5. Explained procedure and purpose to client. Medicated client as needed (i.e., to liquify secretions).			
6. Had client urinate. Determined when client last ate (i.e., waited at least 1 hour past last meal to perform chest P-T).			
7. Instructed client to let therapist know if he/she experiences nausea, chest pain or increasing dyspnea.			
8. Put on protective gear if needed.			
Performing Postural Drainage			
9. Loosened client's clothing. Provided tissues and sputum collection container.			
10. Placed client in proper position for effective drainage of lung segment. Bolstered client with pillows, and covered exposed areas.			
11. Had client maintain position for 5 minutes. Raised side rail if needed.			
12. Encouraged client to cough and expectorate secretions following positioning.			
13. Increased duration time for positioning in subsequent treatments (i.e., up to 15 minutes).			

	S	U	COMMENTS
Performing Percussion			
14. Raised bed to comfortable working height and stood on opposite side of chest area to be percussed.			
15. Cupped hands and clapped rhythmically with alternating hands onto affected area of chest for 3 minutes.			
16. Encouraged client to cough and expectorate following percussion.			
Performing Vibration			
17. Instructed client to inhale slowly and deeply through nose and to exhale through pursed lips during the treatment.			
18. Flattened hands and placed them over affected area of client's chest.			
19. Gently vibrated hands over chest area as client exhaled.			
20. Encouraged client to cough and expectorate following vibration.			
All Chest P-T			
21. Reassessed client condition following chest P-T.			
22. Repeated chest P-T for each affected lung segment.			
23. Slowly returned bed to normal position and assisted client to position of comfort.			
24. Provided oral hygiene and had client wash hands.			
25. Lowered bed and raised side rails if needed.			
26. Discarded protective gear and washed hands.			
27. Reassessed client's condition (i.e., HR and rhythm and quality of secretions).			
28. Documented the procedure in client's record, including assessment data and client response.			

Name _____   Specific Skill Performed _____

Date _____   Attempt Number _____

Instructor _____   PASS _____   FAIL _____

PERFORMANCE CHECKLIST 17.9   INSERTING AN ORAL AIRWAY

	S	U	COMMENTS
1. Assessed client condition and determined need.			
2. Obtained correct size airway and other needed equipment.			
3. Explained procedure and purpose to client/family.			
4. Put on gloves and raised bed to comfortable working height.			
5. Placed client in supine position (semi-Fowler's can be used) and hyperextended neck/head backwards if not contraindicated.			
6. Asked client to open mouth (or opened mouth if client unable).			
7. Held oral airway in horizontal position and inserted it until it touched back of oropharynx. Then gently rotated it downwards (until flat against tongue).			
8. Checked for proper placement of airway. Secured it with tape.			
9. Suctioned oral cavity if needed and cleaned client's face.			
10. Removed gloves and washed hands. Lowered bed.			
11. Reassessed client's condition.			
12. Documented the procedure including assessment data and client response.			

Additional Comments:

_____

_____

_____

_____

_____

_____

_____

_____

Name _____   Specific Skill Performed _____

Date _____   Attempt Number _____

Instructor _____   PASS _____   FAIL _____

PERFORMANCE CHECKLIST 17.10 **SUCTIONING THE OROPHARYNGEAL CAVITY**

	S	U	COMMENTS
1. Assessed client condition and determined need.			
2. Reviewed chart to determine position of sutures/trauma if appropriate.			
3. Gathered appropriate equipment.			
4. Explained procedure and purpose to client/family.			
5. Placed cup of water in convenient location and prepared other equipment for use (i.e., attached suction tip, tubing and suction unit, turned on suction, etc.).			
6. Raised bed to comfortable working height, lowered side rail and assisted client to position that allowed accessibility to oral cavity. Protected client's clothing with towel placed across chest.			
7. Put on gloves and other protective gear as needed.			
8. Inspected/observed client's oral/pharnygeal cavity.			
9. Tested capability of the suctioning apparatus before beginning the procedure.			
10. Removed oxygen mask from client's face if present.			
11. Gently inserted tip (with suction occluded) along client's gum line to back of oral cavity.			
12. Applied suction and removed secretions. Encouraged client to cough if appropriate.			
13. Removed suction device and replaced oxygen mask.			
14. Rinsed suction tip by suctioning water from cup.			
15. Reassessed client condition and resuctioned if needed. Replaced oxygen after each suctioning attempt.			
16. When suctioning completed, turned off suction. Cleaned the tip and stored it appropriately. Discarded cup.			
17. Cleaned client's face and assisted client to position of comfort.			

	S	U	COMMENTS
18. Removed gloves. Washed hands.			
19. Reassessed client's condition and oral cavity.			
20. Lowered bed and raised side rails if needed.			
21. Documented the procedure including assessment data and client response.			

Additional Comments:

_____

_____

_____

_____

_____

_____

_____

_____

_____

_____

_____

_____

_____

_____

_____

_____

_____

_____

Name _____   Specific Skill Performed _____

Date _____   Attempt Number _____

Instructor _____   PASS _____   FAIL _____

PERFORMANCE CHECKLIST 17.11 SUCTIONING AN INFANT WITH A BULB SYRINGE

	S	U	COMMENTS
1. Assessed child's respiratory status and determined need for suctioning.			
2. Collected equipment and placed for easy accessibility.			
3. Explained procedure and purpose to child/family.			
4. Put on gloves.			
5. Appropriately positioned and restrained child (i.e., cradled in arm, papoosed, or held lightly in place by therapist's upper torso).			
6. Placed cloth across chest. Placed tissues nearby.			
7. With dominant hand, held/compressed bulb syringe until air expelled.			
8. Gently inserted tip of syringe into child's mouth or nares and gradually released the pressure.			
9. After pressure released (and secretions drawn into bulb syringe), removed syringe and discharged contents into tissue.			
10. Reassessed child's respiratory status and resuctioned if necessary. Allowed child to take several breaths between suctioning attempts and stopped if child's condition worsened.			
11. When suctioning completed, cleaned child's face. Removed restrains and provided comfort. Positioned child to allow for ease of respiration.			
12. Discarded tissues. Cleaned and stored the bulb syringe according to agency policy. Placed linens in appropriate place.			
13. Removed gloves and washed hands.			
14. Reassessed child's respiratory status.			
15. Documented the procedure including assessment data and client response.			

PERFORMANCE CHECKLIST 17.12 **TRACHEOBRONCHIAL SUCTIONING VIA THE NASOTRACHEAL, ENDOTRACHEAL, AND TRACHEOSTOMY ROUTES**

	S	U	COMMENTS
1. Assessed client's respiratory status and determined need.			
2. Assembled equipment/supplies and placed for easy accessibility. Solicited help if needed.			
3. Explained procedure and purpose to client/family.			
4. Raised bed, lowered side rail and assisted client to semi-Fowler's position.			
5. Attached tubing to suction apparatus (if not already done) and turned on suction.			
6. Protected client's clothing with towel and inserted airway if appropriate (i.e., if nasotracheal suction needed).			
7. Washed hands and put on mask/goggles/gown if needed.			
8. Prepared suction kit and/or other equipment for use and put on sterile gloves.			
9. Maintained sterile technique during setup and did not contaminate dominant hand when connecting the suction catheter to the tubing.			
10. Had client take several deep breaths prior to suctioning. If client on ventilator, hyperinflated lungs (i.e., sigh) or had assistant hyperinflate lungs with ambu-bag. If assistant not available, disconnected tubing (i.e., ventilator) with non-dominant hand after hyperinflation.			
11. Used sterile dominant hand to insert catheter.			
12. Suctioned client via appropriate route (see following routes).			
Suctioning via the Nasotracheal Route			
13. Inserted/advanced catheter through nose (without suction) as client inhaled until resistance met, cough stimulated, or secretions reached.			

	S	U	COMMENTS
14. Rotated catheter and applied intermittent suction as catheter withdrawn.			
15. Did not suction longer than 10 to 15 seconds.			
Suctioning via the Endotracheal Route			
16. Quickly inserted/advanced catheter (without suction) through client's endotracheal tube during inspiration until resistance met, cough stimulated or secretions found.			
17. Rotated catheter and applied intermittent suction as catheter withdrawn. Asked client to cough if able.			
18. Did not suction longer than 10 to 15 seconds.			
19. Replaced (or assistant replaced) oxygen source and hyperinflated client's lungs with 5 deep breaths (ambu-bag or ventilator) or had client take deep breaths if appropriate.			
20. Rinsed catheter with saline suctioned from cup.			
21. Waited one minute before repeating steps 16-19 (with fresh suction kit) if additional suction needed.			
22. Assessed client's respiratory status between suctioning attempts.			
23. Replaced ventilator, oxygen or humidification device.			
Suctioning via the Tracheostomy Route			
24. Quickly inserted/advanced catheter (without suction) through client's endotrachael tube during inspiration until resistance met, cough stimulated, or secretions found.			
25. Rotated catheter and applied intermittent suction as catheter withdrawn. Asked client to cough if able.			
26. Did not suction longer than 10 to 15 seconds.			
27. Replaced (or assistant replaced) oxygen source and hyperinflated client's lungs with 5 deep breaths (ambu-bag or ventilator) or had client take deep breaths if appropriate.			
28. Rinsed catheter with saline suctioned from cup.			
29. Waited one minute before repeating steps 24-27 (with fresh suction kit) if additional suction needed.			

	S	U	COMMENTS
30. Assessed client's respiratory status between suctioning attempts.			
31. Replaced ventilator, oxygen or humidification device.			
32. Referred to Performance Checklist 17.13 if tracheostomy care/ cleaning needed.			
33. Suctioned oral and nasal cavities after tracheobronchial airway cleared of secretions.			
34. Appropriately removed catheter (i.e., rolled inside glove) and discarded according to agency policy.			
35. Used remaining gloved hand to discard/clean other equipment/ supplies. Removed/discarded glove.			
36. Put on exam gloves and provided oral hygiene to client. Checked to be sure that cuff (i.e., endotracheal or tracheostomy) was properly inflated before giving oral hygiene. Changed ties/tape if appropriate.			
37. Positioned client for comfort, put up side rails and lowered bed.			
38. Discarded gloves and washed hands.			
39. Reassessed client's condition.			
40. Documented procedure including assessment data and client response.			

Additional Comments:

_____

_____

_____

_____

_____

_____

_____

_____

Name _____   Specific Skill Performed _____
Date _____   Attempt Number _____
Instructor _____   PASS _____   FAIL _____

PERFORMANCE CHECKLIST 17.13 CARING FOR A CLIENT WITH A TRACHEOSTOMY

	S	U	COMMENTS
1. Assessed client's respiratory status and determined meed for suctioning and tracheostomy care.			
2. Gathered appropriate equipment/supplies and placed them for easy accessibility. Solicited help if needed.			
3. Explained procedure and purpose to client/family.			
4. Raised bed, lowered side rail, assisted client to semi-Fowler's position (side-lying if unconscious) and placed towel across client's chest.			
5. Placed end of suction tubing within easy reach and turned on suction.			
6. Opened suction kit and prepared it for use (i.e., added saline to cups).			
7. Prepared sterile field and added tracheostomy cleaning supplies (i.e., sterile containers with hydrogen peroxide and saline, brush, swabs, gauzes, etc.). Opened disposable inner cannula if appropriate. Did not contaminate supplies.			
8. Prepared correct length of new tape for tracheostomy necktie.			
9. Put on gown, mask and goggles if needed.			
10. Put on sterile gloves and suctioned client (see Performance Checklist 17.12).			
11. Removed tracheostomy bib (drain sponge) and discarded it.			
12. Discarded soiled gloves. Re-gloved with new sterile gloves. Kept dominant hand sterile through rest of procedure.			
13. Replaced or removed/cleaned the inner cannula.			
Replacing Disposable Inner Cannula			
14. With non-dominant hand unlocked and removed the inner cannula.			
15. Resuctioned client if needed.			

	S	U	COMMENTS
16. With dominant hand, picked up new inner cannula and moistened it with saline.			
17. Inserted inner cannula into outer cannula and locked it into place.			
18. Reattached oxygen source.			

Cleaning a Non-disposable Inner Cannula

	S	U	COMMENTS
19. Removed inner cannula with non-dominant hand and placed it in container of hydrogen proxide.			
20. Placed oxygen source close to tracheostomy (or had assistant maintain ventilation with ambu-bag if needed) during cleaning process.			
21. Cleaned inner cannula with hydrogen peroxide and brush. Rinsed well with saline and drained off excess. Reinserted inner cannula and locked it into place.			
22. Reattached oxygen source.			

Cleaning the Tracheostomy Stoma

	S	U	COMMENTS
23. Cleaned around stoma, outer surfaces of tube and the surrounding skin with hydrogen peroxide (i.e., gauze and swabs). Cleaned from the stoma outwards.			
24. Rinsed the same areas with saline (i.e., gauze and swabs) and patted with dry gauze.			

Changing the Trachestomy Necktie

	S	U	COMMENTS
25. Left old necktie in place while putting on new one (unless assistant available to hold cannula in).			
26. Threaded new tie through one side of face plate and brought both ends around back of client's neck to other side of face plate.			
27. Threaded one free end through the other sides of the face plate and tied the ends together firmly but not tightly.			
28. Cut away/removed old necktie and discarded.			
29. Placed a clean tracheostomy bib on dressing around outer cannula under trach ties and face plate.			

	S	U	COMMENTS
30. Suctioned client again if necessary (see Performance Checklist 17.12).			
31. Replaced oxygen source.			
32. Provided oral care (with cuff inflated if present).			
33. Disposed of soiled equipment appropriately. Discarded gloves.			

Deflating and Inflating an Airway Tube Cuff

	S	U	COMMENTS
34. Put on gloves and suctioned the oropharyngeal cavity.			
35. Released clamp if present and attached syringe to inflation tube.			
36. Slowly withdrew air from cuff as client inhaled (or ventilated by assistant with ambu-bag).			
37. Observed for respiratory difficulties.			

Inflating Airway Tube Cuff Using Minimal Occlusive Volume (MOV) and Minimal Leak Technique (MLT)

	S	U	COMMENTS
38. Placed stethoscope on client's neck and listened during cuff inflation.			
39. Inflated cuff with syringe. Used smallest amount of air needed to obtain a seal (2 to 5 ml.).			
40. Aspirated small amount of air (0.1 to 3 ml.) back into syringe until a very slight air leak is heard.			
41. Noted the total amount of air inserted into cuff. Clamped tube if necessary and removed syringe.			
42. Measured cuff pressure with manometer if available.			
43. Documented procedure including time of deflation, amount of air reinserted, client response, and measurement of cuff pressure.			

Completion of Care

	S	U	COMMENTS
44. Positioned client for comfort, raised side rails and lowered bed.			
45. Removed gloves and washed hands.			
46. Reassessed client's condition.			

	S	U	COMMENTS
47. Documented the procedure including assessment data and client response.			
49. Obtained additional supplies (if needed) to be placed at bedside.			

Additional Comments:

_____

_____

_____

_____

_____

_____

_____

_____

_____

_____

_____

_____

_____

_____

_____

_____

_____

_____

_____

_____

Name _____   Specific Skill Performed _____
Date _____   Attempt Number _____
Instructor _____   PASS _____   FAIL _____

PERFORMANCE CHECKLIST 17.14 PROVIDING ENDOTRACHEAL TUBE CARE

	S	U	COMMENTS
1. Assessed client's respiratory status and determined need for suctioning and endotracheal tube.			
2. Gathered appropriate equipment/supplies and placed them for easy accessibility. Solicited help if needed.			
3. Explained procedure and purpose to client/family.			
4. Raised bed, lowered side rail, assisted client to semi-Fowler's position (side-lying if unconscious) and placed towel across client's chest.			
5. Placed end of suction tubing within easy reach and turned on suction.			
6. Opened suction kit and prepared it for use (i.e., added saline to cups).			
7. Prepared equipment/supplies for oral hygiene (i.e., soap, water, washcloths, etc), oral airway cleaning (i.e., hydrogen peroxide, brush), and endotracheal tube cleaning (i.e., adhesive remover).			
8. Prepared replacement tape/tie (i.e., adhesive tape strap or twill tape tie and placed it for easy accessibility).			
9. Checked to see that all needed equipment was ready.			
10. Opened suction kit, put on gloves and suctioned client (see Performance Checklist 17.12).			
11. While client was being re-oxygenated (i.e., on ventilator or by assistant with ambu-bag), checked again to ascertain that all needed equipment was available including additional suctioning equipment (i.e., oral and endotracheal).			
12. Had gloved assistant hold the ET tube firmly in place at client's lip line without disturbing client's respirations (i.e., oxygen source attached and client continuously ventilated).			
13. Removed tape from around ET tube, client's skin, and discarded. Used adhesive remover if needed.			
14. Removed oral airway (or bite block) and placed it in hydrogen peroxide.			

	S	U	COMMENTS
15. Performed oral hygiene appropriate for the type airway present (i.e., nasotracheal or orotracheal). If orotracheal tube in place, performed oral care on one side then had assistant move tube to other side of mouth so remaining area could be cleaned. Checked to see that reference mark on ET tube remained at the same level.			
16. Bathed client's face and neck and provided facial shave if appropriate.			
17. Secured ET tube with prepared adhesive straps or twill tape.			
Securing ET tube with Adhesive Tape			
18. Brushed attachment area on face with tincture of benzoin and let dry.			
19. Auscultated lungs. Checked for bilateral breath sounds in all lung fields.			
20. Slid prepared adhesive strap under neck (sticky side up and non-adherent part under neck).			
21. Attached sticky part of tape (from ear to ET tube) on one side of client's face, split remaining tape lengthwise, and correctly wrapped around ET tube to secure it.			
22. Pulled adhesive strap snugly around neck (i.e., not tight but leaving no excess) and secured other side of ET tube in same manner.			
Securing ET Tube With Twill Tape			
23. Placed doubled-over 2-foot twill tape around ET tube and brought ends through loop.			
24. Checked placement of tape on tube (i.e., below mark of where ET leaves mouth or nose) and tied the tape tightly to the tube.			
25. Pulled the tape ends in opposite directions around and behind neck and tied in a secure knot at side of client's neck. Checked to be sure that the tape around neck was snug but not tight.			
Completion of Care			
26. Ascertained that attachments to ventilator/oxygen source were secure.			

	S	U	COMMENTS
27. Cleaned oral airway with peroxide, rinsed well and reinserted.			
28. Positioned client for comfort, raised side rails and lowered bed.			
29. Disposed of equipment according to agency guidelines.			
30. Removed gloves, washed hands and put away left-over supplies. Left one suction kit for easy accessibility.			
31. Reassessed client condition (i.e., cardiac, respiratory, comfort).			
32. Documented procedure including assessment data and client response.			
33. Obtained additional supplies if needed and stored in client's room.			

Additional Comments:

_____

_____

_____

_____

_____

_____

_____

_____

_____

_____

_____

_____

_____

_____

_____

_____

Name _____   Specific Skill Performed _____

Date _____   Attempt Number _____

Instructor _____   PASS _____   FAIL _____

PERFORMANCE CHECKLIST 17.15 MANAGING A CHEST TUBE

	S	U	COMMENTS
Preparing for Insertion of a Chest Tube			
1. Assessed client's respiratory and cardiac status.			
2. Checked chart for physician's order/rationale for chest tube (CT) and determined drainage system to be used. Checked for signed consent form if appropriate.			
3. Obtained appropriate equipment and took to beside if procedure to be done in client's room.			
4. Explained procedure and purpose to client/family.			
5. Placed chest tube insertion tray for easy access by physician.			
6. Prepared the drainage system. Maintained sterile technique throughout setup.			
Using a One-Bottle System Setup			
7. Removed cover from vent of sterile vented water-seal chest tube bottle.			
8. Added enough sterile water or saline to bottle to cover bottom of longer tube by 1" (2 cm.). Did not contaminate system.			
9. Assessed integrity of system.			
Using a Two-Bottle System Setup			
10. Set up a sterile water-seal bottle (Bottle #2) as above (i.e., as for one-bottle system).			
11. Used a sterile connector rod to attach the vent opening of the sterile drainage collection bottle (Bottle #1) to the submerged longer tube of the water-seal bottle (Bottle #2).			
12. Left the non-submerged tube on water-seal bottle open to air.			
13. Did not contaminate system and did not remove cover from second tube in drainage bottle (i.e., vent for chest tube connection after insertion).			

	S	U	COMMENTS
14. Assessed integrity of system.			
Using a Three-Bottle System Setup			
15. Set up a water-seal bottle (Bottle #2) and a drainage collection bottle (Bottle #1) as above.			
16. Added enough sterile water or saline to sterile suction control bottle (Bottle #3) to cover longer tube with 1" (2 cm.) of fluid. Left other end of long tube open to air.			
17. Used second connector rod to attach the vent opening (short tube) on water-seal bottle (Bottle #2) to one of the short tubes on suction control bottle (Bottle #3).			
18. Connected the second short tube on suction control bottle to suction source.			
19. Did not remove cover from client's chest tube connection or drainage bottle (Bottle #1).			
20. Assessed integrity of system.			
Using a Disposable System			
21. Followed manufacturer's directions to set up system.			
22. Placed a strip of adhesive tape vertically on collection bottle next to calibrated numbers.			
Assisting with Insertion of Chest Tube			
23. Provided privacy. Raised bed, lowered side rail and assisted client to Fowler's or semi-Fowler's position.			
24. Put on gloves and prepped the insertion site. Shaved site if necessary. Discarded gloves.			
25. Put on sterile gloves and assisted physician as needed.			
26. Monitored client's condition (i.e., cardiac, respiratory, psychologic status) during procedure.			
27. After CT insertion, connected distal end of chest tube(s) to functional drainage system. Used "Y" connector to connect CT to drainage system if 2 CTs are used.			

	S	U	COMMENTS
28. Checked to see that all connections were tight and secured them with adhesive tape.			
29. Disposed of equipment appropriately.			
30. Removed gloves and washed hands.			
31. Assisted client in semi-to-high Fowler's position (if tolerated) and reassessed client's condition.			
32. Raised side rail and lowered bed.			
33. Timed and dated the collection bottle and noted the amount and characteristics of the drainage. Noted presence of bubbling in collection bottle/chamber.			
34. Documented the procedure including assessment data, amount and characteristics of drainage, amount suction applied and client response.			
35. Periodically monitored client for development of tension pneumothorax and took appropriate steps if needed (i.e., examined CT for occlusion and notified physician). (See step 39 below).			
36. Examined and recorded the chest tube drainage (i.e., on tape strip and in client record) according to agency protocol (i.e., q 1° post-op and/or large amount drainage, q 8° for all clients with CT).			
Monitoring the Client with a Chest Tube			
37. Ensured that necessary equipment was at client's bedside in case of emergency (i.e., rubber-shod Kelly clamp, sterile petrolatum gauze dressing, extra drainage system.).			
38. Periodically ascertained that: a. Connections were secure. b. Drainage system below CT insertion site. c. Tubing straight without kinks. d. Levels in water-seal bottle/chamber at proper mark. e. Suction level maintained as ordered (i.e., gentle, continuous bubbling). f. Drainage did not collect in tube. g. Air leaks were not present. h. Drainage bottle/chamber not filled/overfilled.			

	S	U	COMMENTS
39. If drainage collects in tubing (i.e., sluggish drainage or impeded/occluded by clots) checked for occlusion and notified physician. Followed agency protocol/guidelines for "milking" chest tube if physician ordered it done. Did not occlude CT for more than one minute during milking process if done.			
40. If air leak present (i.e., continuous bubbling in the water-seal bottle/chamber), checked for location of leak by occluding CT near client's chest with rubber-shod Kelly clamps. Did not leave clamps in place longer than one minute. a. If leak in drainage system (i.e., bubbling continued with clamps in place), checked integrity of connections and retaped them. Replaced drainage system if necessary.			
b. If leak at chest tube insertion site (i.e., bubbling stopped with clamps in place), reinforced the occlusive chest dressing. Notified physician if leak continued.			
41. If drainage bottle/chamber full, set up new drainage system, put on gloves and replaced old system with new one. Clamped CT just long enough to disconnect old/connect new drainage system. Checked integrity of new system and reassessed client condition.			
42. Documented any trouble-shooting activities/procedures including assessment data, and client response.			

Additional Comments:

_____

_____

_____

_____

_____

_____

_____

_____

_____

_____

_____

_____

_____

Name _____   Specific Skill Performed _____

Date _____   Attempt Number _____

Instructor _____   PASS _____   FAIL _____

PERFORMANCE CHECKLIST 18.1 APPLYING MEDICATIONS TO THE SKIN

	S	U	COMMENTS
1. Checked client's chart for physician's order, rationale for medication and client drug allergies.			
2. Washed hands. Focused attention on medication preparation.			
3. Obtained correct medication, read label, and checked expiration date.			
4. Checked medication label again and placed it on tray with other equipment if needed (i.e., applicator, dressing, tape, etc.).			
5. Took medication/equipment to client and introduced self.			
6. Verified client's identity (i.e., checked arm band, read bed tag, and asked client to state name).			
7. Inquired about drug allergies.			
8. Explained about medication and its purpose.			
9. Checked medication label for third time.			
10. Provided privacy and positioned client appropriately for application of medication. Exposed/draped application site.			
11. Put on gloves.			
12. Put linen protector under body part if needed.			
13. Appropriately cleaned and dried area to be treated.			
14. Assessed condition of clients skin (i.e., color, temperature, circulation, drainage, texture, etc.).			
15. Changed gloves if necessary.			
16. Correctly administered the medication.			
17. **Administering an Aerosol Spray**			
a. Shook container well and followed manufacturer's instructions regarding application (i.e., distance from which to spray, etc.).			

	S	U	COMMENTS
b. Sprayed medication evenly over area. Did not direct spray toward client's face.			
18. Administering Creams, Gels, Pastes, Ointments and Oil-Based Lotions			
a. Placed 1 to 2 tsps. of medication in palm of gloved hand (or used tongue blade).			
b. Applied medication evenly and smoothly over affected area.			
19. Administering Nitroglycerine Paste or Ointment			
a. Squeezed out ordered amount of paste onto paper measuring guide.			
b. Removed old patch and discarded. Cleansed skin.			
c. Placed new ointment and paper on skin in a different location from old patch. Avoided hairy areas. Did not touch ointment.			
d. Taped the patch in place according to agency protocol (i.e., cover with plastic wrap, etc.).			
20. Applying a Transdermal Patch			
a. Removed backing from patch according to manufacturer's directions and applied patch to smooth skin area.			
b. Removed old patch and discarded.			
21. Applying Suspension-based Lotions			
a. Shook medication well.			
b. Moistened gauze pad or cotton ball with lotion and patted onto affected area.			
22. Applying Powders			
a. Checked to see that area was dry.			
b. Dusted area lightly with powder.			
23. Applying Liniments			
a. Poured 1 to 2 tsps. of liniment into gloved hand.			
b. Applied to client's skin in smooth, even strokes.			

	S	U	COMMENTS
After Administration of Medication			
24. Placed dressing over affected area if appropriate.			
25. Replaced clothing and assisted client to position of comfort.			
26. Disposed of soiled supplies.			
27. Removed gloves and washed hands.			
28. Checked on effects of medication at appropriate time.			
29. Documented the application including assessment data and client response if appropriate.			

Additional Comments:

_____

_____

_____

_____

_____

_____

_____

_____

_____

_____

_____

_____

_____

_____

Name _____   Specific Skill Performed _____
Date _____   Attempt Number _____
Instructor _____ PASS _____   FAIL _____

PERFORMANCE CHECKLIST 18.2 ADMINISTERING OPTIC MEDICATIONS

		S	U	COMMENTS
1.	Checked client's chart for physician's orders, rationale for medication and client drug allergies.			
2.	Washed hands. Focused attention on medication preparation.			
3.	Obtained correct medication, read label, and checked expiration date.			
4.	Checked medication label again and placed it on tray with other equipment if needed (i.e., applicators, dressing, tape, etc.).			
5.	Took medication/equipment to client and introduced self.			
6.	Verified client's identity (i.e., checked arm band, read bed tag, and asked client to state name).			
7.	Inquired about drug allergies.			
8.	Explained about medication and its purpose.			
9.	Checked medication label for third time.			
10.	Provided privacy if needed and positioned client (supine or in chair) with head hyperextended.			
11.	Put on sterile gloves.			
12.	Appropriately cleaned client's eye(s).			
13.	Assessed condition of eye (i.e., redness, drainage, lesions, etc.)			
14.	Changed gloves if needed.			
15.	Provided tissue for client to hold just below the lower eyelid. Removed/loosened cap on medication container.			
16.	Used non-dominant hand to correctly open client's eye and expose conjunctival sac.			
17.	Asked client to look up and try not to blink.			
18.	Correctly administered the medication.			

	S	U	COMMENTS
19. Instilling Eye Drops			
a. Used dominant hand (resting on client's forehead) to hold dropper 1/2 inch from sac and instilled prescribed number of drops.			
b. Applied gentle pressure to nasolacrimal duct for one minute if appropriate before allowing client to close eye.			
20. Administering Eye Ointment			
a. Applied thin line of ointment along lower eyelid inside conjunctival sac (from inner canthus to outer).			
b. Asked client to close eye and move eyeball around to spread ointment.			
c. Gently wiped excess medication away.			
21. Applied eye patch if indicated.			
22. Appropriately disposed of soiled supplies.			
23. Removed gloves and washed hands.			
24. Checked on effects of medication at proper time.			
25. Documented the application including assessment data and client response if appropriate.			

Additional Comments:

_____

_____

_____

_____

_____

_____

_____

_____

Name _____   Specific Skill Performed _____

Date _____   Attempt Number _____

Instructor _____   PASS _____   FAIL _____

PERFORMANCE CHECKLIST 18.3   ADMINISTERING OTIC MEDICATION

	S	U	COMMENTS
1. Checked client's chart for physician's order, rationale for medication and client drug allergies.			
2. Washed hands. Focused attention on medication preparation.			
3. Obtained correct medication, read label, and checked expiration date.			
4. Checked medication label again and placed it on tray with other equipment if needed (i.e., applicators, dressing, tape, etc.).			
5. Took medication/equipment to client and introduced self.			
6. Verified client's identity (i.e., checked arm band, read bed tag, and asked client to state name).			
7. Inquired about drug allergies.			
8. Explained about medication and its purpose.			
9. Checked medication label for third time.			
10. Assisted client to side-lying position with affected ear upwards.			
11. Put on gloves.			
12. Assessed client's external ear for drainage/inflammation and inquired about pain.			
13. Gently cleaned away drainage or cerumen but did not push applicator into ear canal.			
14. With non-dominant hand, grasped client's ear and pulled to straighten ear canal (i.e., for adult, up and out; for child, down and out.			
15. With dominant hand resting on forehead, held medicine dropper 1/2" above ear and instilled prescribed number of drops. Did not touch dropper to ear or anything else.			
16. Applied gentle pressure to tragus of ear, then placed a small cotton ball into external ear canal if appropriate.			
17. Instructed client to remain on side for 2 to 3 minutes and remove cotton ball after 10 to 15 minutes.			

	S	U	COMMENTS
18. Assisted client to sitting position if needed.			
19. Disposed of soiled supplies appropriately.			
20. Removed gloves and washed hands.			
21. Checked on effects of medication at proper time.			
22. Documented the application including assessment data and client response if appropriate.			

Additional Comments:

_____

_____

_____

_____

_____

_____

_____

_____

_____

_____

_____

_____

_____

_____

_____

_____

_____

_____

_____

Name _____   Specific Skill Performed _____

Date _____   Attempt Number _____

Instructor _____   PASS _____   FAIL _____

PERFORMANCE CHECKLIST 18.4 ADMINISTERING INHALED MEDICATIONS WITH A METERED-DOSE INHALER

	S	U	COMMENTS
1. Checked client's chart for physician's orders, rationale for medication and client drug allergies.			
2. Washed hands. Focused attention on medication preparation.			
3. Obtained correct medication, read label, and checked expiration date.			
4. Checked medication label again and placed it on tray with other equipment if needed (i.e., applicator, dressing, tape, etc.).			
5. Took medication/equipment to client and introduced self.			
6. Verified client's identity (i.e., checked arm band, read bed tag, and asked client to state name).			
7. Inquired about drug allergies.			
8. Explained about medication and its purpose.			
9. Checked medication label for third time.			
10. Assessed client's condition (i.e., cardiac, respiratory) including ability to hold and manipulate inhalation device.			
11. Had client self-administer the medication if possible. Assessed client's ability to administer medication. a. Put mouthpiece in mouth. b. Exhale deeply through nose. c. Simultaneously depress inhalation device and inhale deeply through mouth. d. Hold breath for several seconds. e. Exhale slowly through pursed lips.			
12. Assisted with administration of med if necessary.			
13. Assessed client's respiratory status (i.e., for wheezing) and cardiac status (i.e., cardiac dysrhythmia) following administration of medication.			
14. Documented the application including assessment data, client response and any teaching-learning activities.			

PERFORMANCE CHECKLIST 18.5 ADMINISTERING NASAL INSTILLATIONS

	S	U	COMMENTS
1. Checked client's chart for physician's order, rationale for medication, and client drug allergies.			
2. Washed hands. Focused attention on medication preparation.			
3. Obtained correct medication, read label, and checked expiration date.			
4. Checked medication label again and placed it on tray with other equipment if needed (i.e., applicator, dressing, tape, etc.).			
5. Took medication/equipment to client and introduced self.			
6. Verified client's identity (i.e., checked arm band, read bed tag, and asked client to state name).			
7. Inquired about drug allergies.			
8. Explained about medication, purpose, and what to expect.			
9. Checked medication label for third time.			
10. Assessed client for breathing obstruction, pain/discomfort, discharge, redness and/or encrustations.			

Instilling Drops

	S	U	COMMENTS
11. Had client blow nose and inspected discharge.			
12. Assisted client to correct position and explained purpose for it.			
13. Drew up correct dosage in dropper.			
14. Had client breathe through mouth while drops were being instilled.			
15. Used appropriate technique to instill drops and did not contaminate dropper.			
16. Had client remain in position for 5 minutes.			

	S	U	COMMENTS
Instilling Sprays			
17. Had client exhale, close one nostril, and then inhale during instillation of spray into other nostril.			
18. Provided tissue to blot excess spray but cautioned client not to blow nose.			
After Administration of Medication			
19. Assisted client to position of comfort.			
20. Discarded soiled supplies.			
21. Reassessed client after 15 to 30 minutes for response to medication.			
22. Documented the application including assessment data and client response.			

Additional Comments:

_____

_____

_____

_____

_____

_____

_____

_____

_____

_____

_____

_____

_____

_____

_____

Name _____   Specific Skill Performed _____

Date _____   Attempt Number _____

Instructor _____   PASS _____   FAIL _____

PERFORMANCE CHECKLIST 18.6 ADMINISTERING RECTAL MEDICATIONS

	S	U	COMMENTS
1. Checked client's chart for physician's order, rationale for medication and client drug allergies.			
2. Washed hands. Focused attention on medication preparation.			
3. Obtained correct medication, read label, and checked expiration date.			
4. Checked medication label again and placed it on tray with other equipment if needed (i.e., applicator, dressing, tape, etc.).			
5. Took medication/equipment to client and introduced self.			
6. Verified client's identity (i.e., checked arm band, read bed tag, and asked client to state name).			
7. Inquired about drug allergies.			
8. Explained about medication and purpose.			
9. Checked medication label for third time.			
10. Asked when client had last BM and determined if small enema needed before suppository inserted.			
11. Provided privacy, raised bed, lowered rail, assisted client to left lateral position with right leg flexed and positioned self facing client's back.			
12. Opened wrapper but left suppository on it and laid aside.			
13. Put water-soluble lubricant on paper towel and placed it for convenient use.			
14. Put on glove(s).			
15. Separated client's buttocks and inspected area for hemorrhoids or bleeding.			
16. Lubricated suppository and index finger of dominant hand.			
17. Asked client to breathe through mouth while suppository is inserted.			

	S	U	COMMENTS
18. Gently inserted suppository against rectal mucosa (adult 4", child 2").			
19. After insertion, held client's buttocks together for a short while and asked client to retain suppository for specified amount of time.			
20. Discarded gloves and washed hands.			
21. Assisted client to position of comfort with bed lowered and call light within easy reach.			
22. Reassessed client after specified time to check for results.			
23. Documented the application including assessment data and client response.			

Additional Comments:

_____

_____

_____

_____

_____

_____

_____

_____

_____

_____

_____

_____

_____

_____

_____

_____

Name _____   Specific Skill Performed _____
Date _____   Attempt Number _____
Instructor _____   PASS _____   FAIL _____

PERFORMANCE CHECKLIST 18.7 ADMINISTERING VAGINAL MEDICATIONS

	S	U	COMMENTS
1. Checked client's chart for physician's order, rationale for medication and client drug allergies.			
2. Washed hands. Focused attention on medication preparation.			
3. Obtained correct medication, read label, and checked expiration date.			
4. Checked medication label again and placed it on tray with other equipment if needed (i.e., applicator, dressing, tape, etc.).			
5. Took medication/equipment to client and introduced self.			
6. Verified client's identity (i.e., checked arm band, read bed tag, and asked client to state name).			
7. Inquired about drug allergies.			
8. Explained about medication and purpose.			
9. Checked medication label for third time.			
10. Determined if client had procedure done before. If not, explained what can be expected.			
11. Had client void.			
12. Washed hands and arranged supplies for easy accessibility.			
13. Assisted client to bed, provided privacy, raised bed, lowered rail and helped client assume a dorsal-recumbent position. Appropriately draped client.			
14. Adjusted lighting so client's vaginal orifice was well lighted.			
15. Put on gloves.			
16. Correctly administered the medication.			

	S	U	COMMENTS

Inserting a Suppository

	S	U	COMMENTS
17. Removed wrapper from suppository, placed in applicator (if appropriate) and lubricated it.			
18. Gently retracted labia (with non-dominant hand) and inserted tapered end of suppository with index finger (dominant hand) or applicator.			
19. Wiped perineal area (toilet tissue) and applied perineal pad.			
20. Removed gloves (inside out) and discarded.			
21. Instructed client to remain on back for at least 10 minutes.			

Inserting Foam, Jelly or Cream

	S	U	COMMENTS
22. Filled applicator with medication and lubricated it as needed.			
23. Retracted client's labia (with non-dominant hand) and inserted applicator 2 to 3" into vagina (with dominant hand) and pushed plunger to expel medication.			
24. Withdrew plunger and placed on paper towel.			
25. Wiped perineal area and applied perineal pad.			
26. Instructed client to remain on back for at least 10 minutes.			
27. Washed applicator with soap and water, dried it thoroughly and stored for future use.			
28. Removed gloves and washed hands.			

Administering a Vaginal Irrigation (Douche)

	S	U	COMMENTS
29. Warmed douche solution to 105° to 110° (i.e., comfortable to wrist) and filled douche bag.			
30. Assisted client to semi-recumbent position on bedpan.			
31. Purged tubing of air and lubricated tip as needed.			
32. Hung container/bag on IV pole no more than 2 feet above client's hips.			

	S	U	COMMENTS
33. Inserted nozzle (3"), released the clamp and allowed solution to flow into vagina. Rotated nozzle to allow fluid to flow over all mucosa. Followed specific instructions regarding containment of fluid inside vagina.			
34. After irrigation complete, had client sit up and lean forward to expel any remaining liquid.			
35. Washed equipment and stored for future use.			
36. Removed gloves and washed hands.			
37. Inspected clients outer perineal area (i.e., irritation, discharge, etc.).			
38. Inquired about discomfort (pruritis, burning, pain).			
39. Documented the application/procedure including assessment data and client response.			

Additional Comments:

_____

_____

_____

_____

_____

_____

_____

_____

_____

_____

_____

_____

_____

Name _____   Specific Skill Performed _____
Date _____   Attempt Number _____
Instructor _____   PASS _____   FAIL _____

PERFORMANCE CHECKLIST 18.8 **ADMINISTERING ORAL MEDICATIONS**

	S	U	COMMENTS
1. Checked client's chart for physician's orders, rationale for medication and client's drug allergies.			
2. Washed hands. Focused attention on medication preparation.			
3. Obtained correct medication (i.e., from client's compartment in medicine cart), read label, and checked expiration date.			
4. Selected appropriate container for medicine (i.e., souffle cup, plastic medicine cup).			
5. Checked medication label again.			
6. Prepared the medication.			
Administering Tablets or Capsules			
7. Placed correct number of capsules or tablets into bottle cap then transferred them to souffle cup and placed on medication tray. If unit dose is used, obtained correct medication/dosage and placed on tray.			
8. If client has difficulty swallowing, crushed pills and dissolved them or mixed them with small amount of food and obtained spoon/syringe to administer medicine.			
Administering Liquid Medications			
9. Placed plastic med cup on level surface.			
10. Poured correct amount of liquid med into cup. Did not contaminate label of med bottle. Used meniscus as measuring line.			
Oral Medications			
11. Checked med label third time before returning it to shelf.			
12. Took med to client, introduced self and explained presence.			
13. Inquired about drug allergies.			

	S	U	COMMENTS
14. Verified client's identity (i.e., checked name band/bed tag and asked client to state name).			
15. Assisted client to sit up (unless contraindicated) or to side if necessary.			
16. Told client what med was for. Gave client the med and glass of water with which to swallow it down.			
17. Checked to see that client swallowed the medication.			
18. Returned equipment to med room and washed hands.			
19. Reassessed client at appropriate time to check on response to medicine.			
20. Charted the administration, according to agency policy, including assessment data and client response.			

Additional Comments:

_____

_____

_____

_____

_____

_____

_____

_____

_____

_____

_____

_____

_____

_____

PERFORMANCE CHECKLIST 18.9 ADMINISTERING MEDICATION THROUGH A NASOGASTRIC TUBE

	S	U	COMMENTS
1. Checked client's chart for physician's orders, rationale for medication and client's drug allergies.			
2. Washed hands. Focused attention on medication preparation.			
3. Obtained correction medication (i.e., from client's compartment in med tray), read label and checked expiration date.			
4. Selected appropriate container for med (i.e., souffle cup, plastic med cup).			
5. Checked medication label again.			
6. Put correct dose of medication (i.e., tablets) into clean mortar and checked label for third time.			
7. Crushed tablets into fine powder with the pestle and poured it into a plastic med cup.			
8. Added warm water to the powder and mixed it to dissolve the medication (i.e., 5 to 10 ml. water).			
9. Took med to client, introduced self and explained presence.			
10. Inquired about drug allergies.			
11. Verified client's identity (i.e., checked name band and asked client to state name).			
12. Elevated head of bed 30^0 to 45^0 degrees (unless contraindicated).			
13. Placed linen protector between nasogastric tube and client's bed and clothing.			
14. Ensured that equipment to check tube placement was available (i.e., stethoscope and catheter tipped syringe).			
15. Put on gloves.			
16. Checked for proper placement of nasogastric tube before instilling medication (i.e., aspiration of gastric contents, auscultation of air into stomach).			

	S	U	COMMENTS
17. Drew up medication into catheter tipped syringe, ejected air, and injected medication into nasogastric tube.			
18. Injected 30 ml. of water into nasogastric tube after medication given.			
19. Clamped tube for 30 minutes.			
20. Removed gloves and washed hands.			
21. Returned equipment to med room if appropriate.			
22. Returned to client's room at appropriate time to assess effects of medication.			
23. Documented the administration including assessment data, position of nasogastric tube and client response.			

Additional Comments:

_____

_____

_____

_____

_____

_____

_____

_____

_____

_____

_____

_____

_____

_____

_____

Name _____   Specific Skill Performed _____
Date _____   Attempt Number _____
Instructor _____   PASS _____   FAIL _____

PERFORMANCE CHECKLIST 18.10 ADMINISTERING SUBLINGUAL MEDICATIONS

	S	U	COMMENTS
1. Checked client's chart for physician's orders, rationale for medication and client's drug allergies.			
2. Washed hands. Focused attention on medication preparation.			
3. Obtained correct medication (i.e., from client's compartment in med cart), read label and checked expiration date.			
4. Selected appropriate container for med (i.e., souffle cup, plastic med cup).			
5. Checked medication label again.			
6. Poured correct dose into medication cup and placed on med tray. Checked label for the third time.			
7. Took medication to client, introduced self and explained presence.			
8. Verified client's identity (i.e., checked name band/bed tag and had client state name).			
9. Inquired about drug allergies.			
10. Assisted client to upright position (unless contraindicated).			
11. Placed tablet under client's tongue (with gloved fingers if necessary) and instructed client not to swallow.			
12. Waited until tablet dissolved, then returned equipment to med room.			
13. Washed hands.			
14. Returned to client at appropriate time to assess effects of the med.			
15. Documented the administration including assessment data and client response.			

Additional Comments:

_____

_____

_____

Name _____   Specific Skill Performed _____
Date _____   Attempt Number _____
Instructor _____   PASS _____   FAIL _____

PERFORMANCE CHECKLIST 18.11 **WITHDRAWING MEDICATIONS FROM AN AMPULE AND A VIAL**

	S	U	COMMENTS
1. Checked client's chart for physician's order, rationale for medication and client's drug allergies.			
2. Washed hands. Focused attention on medication preparation.			
3. Obtained correct medication (i.e., from client's compartment in med cart), read label and checked expiration date.			
4. Removed syringe from paper cover without contaminating the inside of the paper cover.			
5. Checked label again and withdrew the medication.			
Withdrawing Medication from an Ampule			
6. Disconnected needle from syringe without contaminating it. Placed it inside paper covering for later use and connected filter needle to syringe.			
7. Checked label on ampule again.			
8. Ensured that entire dose of medication was in bottom of ampule (i.e., thumped top of amp until all med in bottom).			
9. Scored one side of the ampule neck if needed.			
10. Placed piece of gauze or alcohol swab around neck of ampule, and snapped top of ampule off at neck.			
11. Held ampule in non-dominant hand and syringe in other hand, inserted needle into ampule and withdrew all of the medication.			
12. Discarded the ampule.			
13. Discarded the filter needle in sharps container and replaced the needle. Maintained sterile technique throughout.			

	S	U	COMMENTS
Withdrawing Medication from a Vial			
14. Removed the protective covering from vial without touching the rubber top. Swabbed top of vial with alcohol if needed (i.e., multiple-dose vial).			
15. Reconstituted med according to directions if needed.			
16. Removed cap from needle, drew air into syringe equal to medication dose and inserted the needle through center of rubber stopper.			
17. Inverted vial, checked to see that needle tip was above the fluid level and then injected the air into the vial.			
18. Adjusted syringe so needle tip was below fluid level and withdrew correct amount of medication.			
19. Removed needle from vial, and expelled air bubbles from syringe (if present).			
20. Replaced needle with new needle and cap.			
21. Labeled vial if appropriate (i.e., multiple-dose vial).			
22. Rechecked prepared dosage/medication for correctness.			
23. Used appropriate technique and protocol to administer the drug (see Performance Checklists 18.12, 18.13 or 18.15).			
24. Documented the administration.			

Additional Comments:

_____

_____

_____

_____

_____

_____

_____

_____

Name _____ Specific Skill Performed _____

Date _____ Attempt Number _____

Instructor _____ PASS _____ FAIL _____

PERFORMANCE CHECKLIST 18.12 ADMINISTERING INTRADERMAL INJECTIONS

	S	U	COMMENTS
1. Checked client's chart for physician's order, rationale for medication and client's drug allergies.			
2. Washed hands. Focused attention on medication preparation.			
3. Obtained correct medication (i.e., from client's compartment in med cart), read label and checked expiration date.			
4. Selected appropriate syringe and needle to administer medication.			
5. Checked label again, withdrew the medication and placed it on the med tray.			
6. Read label third time before discarding container (or replacing it to storage if appropriate).			
7. Took med to client, introduced self and explained presence.			
8. Verified client's identity (i.e., checked name band/bed tag and asked client to state name).			
9. Provided privacy and assisted client to assume correct position to receive the injection.			
10. Put on gloves and used appropriate technique to cleanse the site.			
11. Used non-dominant hand to spread skin taut at injection site.			
12. Used dominant hand to grasp syringe and needle (bevel side up) and carefully inserted needle (at 10 degree angle) superficially into client's skin just until bevel is covered.			
13. Injected the medication and withdrew needle. Did not aspirate and did not massage the site.			
14. Observed for wheal formation at site. Marked site and applied bandage if needed.			
15. Disposed of uncapped needle in sharps container according to agency policy (i.e., sharps box in room or on med cart).			
16. Assisted client to position of comfort.			

	S	U	COMMENTS
17. Discarded gloves and washed hands. Returned equipment to med room.			
18. Returned to client at appropriate time to assure the effect of med.			
19. Documented the administration including assessment data and client response.			

Additional Comments:

_____

_____

_____

_____

_____

_____

_____

_____

_____

_____

_____

_____

_____

_____

_____

_____

_____

Name _____   Specific Skill Performed _____
Date _____   Attempt Number _____
Instructor _____   PASS _____   FAIL _____

PERFORMANCE CHECKLIST 18.13 ADMINISTERING SUBCUTANEOUS INJECTIONS

	S	U	COMMENTS
1. Checked client's chart for physician's order, rationale for medication and client's drug allergies.			
2. Washed hands. Focused attention on medication preparation.			
3. Obtained correct medication (i.e., from client's compartment in med cart), read label and checked expiration date.			
4. Selected appropriate syringe and needle to administer medication.			
5. Checked label again, withdrew the medication and placed it on the med tray.			
6. Read label third time before discarding container (or replacing it to storage if appropriate).			
7. Took med to client, introduced self and explained presence.			
8. Verified client's identity (i.e., checked name band/bed tag and asked client to state name).			
9. Provided privacy and assisted client to assume correct position to receive the injection.			
10. Put on gloves and used appropriate technique to cleanse the site.			
11. Used thumb and index finger of non-dominant hand to bunch up tissue at injection site.			
12. Used dominant hand to grasp syringe and quickly inserted the needle into injection site at angle appropriate for needle length and amount of adipose tissue (i.e., 45° angle).			
13. Aspirated for blood before injecting med into tissue. Withdrew needle if blood detected and applied pressure.			
14. Following injection of medication, withdrew needle and massaged area (if not contraindicated).			
15. Disposed of uncapped needle in sharps container according to agency policy (i.e., sharps box in client's room or on med cart).			
16. Applied bandage if needed and assisted client to position of comfort.			

	S	U	COMMENTS
17. Disposed of gloves, washed hands and returned equipment to med rooms.			
18. Returned to client at appropriate time to assess the effects of the med.			
19. Documented the administration including assessment data and client response.			

Additional Comments:

_____

_____

_____

_____

_____

_____

_____

_____

_____

_____

_____

_____

_____

_____

_____

_____

_____

_____

Name _____

Date _____

Instructor _____

Specific Skill Performed _____

Attempt Number _____

PASS _____   FAIL _____

PERFORMANCE CHECKLIST 18.14 MIXING INSULIN IN A SYRINGE

	S	U	COMMENTS
1. Checked client's chart for physician's order/rationale (i.e., type of insulin, amount, frequency of administration, etc.).			
2. Discussed insulin administration with client (i.e., self-administration and mixing of insulin at home).			
3. Washed hands. Focused attention on medication preparation.			
4. Obtained correct insulin preparations, read labels and checked expiration date.			
5. Obtained appropriate syringe/needle for injection (i.e., insulin syringe) and placed with insulin(s) on clean working surface (i.e., med cart or tabletop).			
6. Cleaned rubber top on both insulin vials with alcohol swab. Checked labels on vials again.			
7. Injected air in long-acting (cloudy) insulin equal to the amount of insulin to be withdrawn. Did not let needle touch the insulin.			
8. Withdrew needle and injected air into short-acting (clear) insulin equal to the amount of insulin to be withdrawn.			
9. With needle still in clear (regular) insulin, inverted vial and withdrew amount of insulin prescribed.			
10. Inserted needle of syringe (with regular insulin in it) into vial of long-acting insulin, inverted vial and withdrew the prescribed amount of insulin.			
11. Withdrew the needle and checked the total amount of insulin in the syringe.			
12. Rechecked labels on insulin vials for third time before replacing to storage.			
13. Appropriately administered the insulin subcutaneously as prescribed (see Performance Checklist 18.13).			
14. Appropriately documented the administration including assessment data and client response.			

Name _____

Date _____

Instructor _____

PERFORMANCE CHECKLIST 18.15 ADMINISTERING INTRAMUSCULAR INJECTIONS

	S	U	COMMENTS
1. Checked client's chart for physician's order, rationale for medication and client's drug allergies.			
2. Washed hands. Focused attention on medication preparation.			
3. Obtained correct medication (i.e., from client's compartment in med cart), read label and checked expiration date.			
4. Selected appropriate syringe and needle to administer medication.			
5. Checked label again, withdrew the medication, placed 0.2 to 0.5 ml. of air to syringe (air lock), and placed it on the med tray.			
6. Read label third time before discarding container (or replacing it to storage if appropriate).			
7. Took med to client, introduced self and explained presence.			
8. Verified client's identity (i.e., checked name band/bed tag and asked client to state name).			
9. Provided privacy and assisted client to assume correct position to receive the injection.			
10. Put on gloves and used appropriate technique to cleanse the site.			
11. Used thumb and index finger of non-dominant hand to spread tissue at injection site.			
12. Used dominant hand to grasp syringe and quickly inserted the length of the needle at a 90° angle into the injection site. (see step 20 if Z-track technique is indicated.)			
13. Aspirated for blood before injecting medicine into tissues Withdrew needle if blood detected and applied pressure.			
14. Following injection of medication, withdrew needle and massaged area (if not contraindicated).			
15. Disposed of uncapped needle in sharps container according to agency policy (i.e., sharps box in client's room or on med cart).			
16. Applied bandage if needed and assisted client to position of comfort.			

	S	U	COMMENTS
17. Disposed of gloves, washed hands and returned equipment to med room.			
18. Returned to client at appropriate time to assess the effects of the medicine.			
19. Documented the administration including assessment data and client response.			

Z-Track Technique for Intramuscular Injections

	S	U	COMMENTS
20. Used Z-track technique for injection if medication was highly irritating to subcutaneous tissues.			
21. Withdrew medicine into syringe, removed the needle and replaced it with a new sterile needle.			
22. Added air lock to syringe.			
23. With non-dominant hand, grasped the skin and tissues over injection site and stretched it to the side 1 to 1 1/2".			
24. With dominant hand, quickly inserted length of needle at 90° angle.			
25. Used thumb of dominant hand to aspirate for blood.			
26. If no blood noted, injected medication while still holding tissue taut to one side.			
27. Maintained traction on skin for 10 seconds (i.e., counted to 10).			
28. Released skin slowly as needle is withdrawn.			
29. Did not massage area.			

Additional Comments:

_____

_____

_____

_____

_____

_____

_____

Name _____ Specific Skill Performed _____

Date _____ Attempt Number _____

Instructor _____ PASS _____ FAIL _____

PERFORMANCE CHECKLIST 18.16 MIXING MEDICATIONS IN A SYRINGE

	S	U	COMMENTS
1. Checked clients chart for physician's order, rationale and drug allergies.			
2. Washed hands. Focused attention on medication preparation.			
3. Obtained medications and checked the labels to ensure correctness.			
4. Ensured that the medications were compatible and that total dosage less than 2.5 ml.			
5. Selected appropriate syringe and needle to administer the medication.			
6. Used alcohol swab(s) to wipe top(s) of medication vials.			
7. Injected air into vial(s) in amount equal to amount of medicine to be withdrawn.			
8. Checked label(s) again before withdrawing medication. Withdrew prescribed amount from one vial.			
9. Used same syringe (with medicine in it) to withdraw prescribed amount from second vial (or ampule). Did not let any of the first medication enter the second vial as medication was withdrawn.			
10. Checked medication labels a third time to ensure correctness of medications and dosages.			
11. Observed syringe for evidence of incompatibility (i.e., cloudiness or precipitation).			
12. Appropriately administered the medication (see Performance Checklists 18.13, 18.15).			
13. Appropriately documented the administration.			

Additional Comments:

_____

_____

_____

Name _____ Specific Skill Performed _____

Date _____ Attempt Number _____

Instructor _____ PASS _____   FAIL _____

PERFORMANCE CHECKLIST 18.17 ADMINISTERING INTRAVENOUS MEDICATIONS

	S	U	COMMENTS
1. Checked client's chart for physician's order/rationale and drug allergies. Checked medicine cards/pharmacology book/pharmacist to verify correctness with MD order.			
2. Verified that secondary medication was compatible with the primary fluid.			
3. Went to client's room and assessed IV site for patency. Inquired about allergies.			
4. Obtained correct medication and read the label. Checked the expiration date.			
5. Checked the label again.			
6. Prepared and administered the medication.			
Administering Intravenous Push Medications			
7. Selected appropriate syringe and needle to prepare medicine.			
8. Used sterile technique while reconstituting and drawing up medicine. Recapped needle.			
9. Checked label for third time.			
10. Took med to client and verified client's identity.			
11. Cleaned IV tubing injection port with alcohol swab.			
12. Inserted syringe needle into injection port and occluded IV tubing above the port with fingers while injecting medication.			
Adding Medication to a Primary Bag			
13. Selected appropriate syringe and needle to prepare medication.			
14. Used sterile technique while reconstituting and drawing up medication. Recapped needle.			
15. Checked label for third time.			

	S	U	COMMENTS
16. Cleaned port of primary bag, inserted needle and injected medication into bag of fluid.			
17. Rotated bag to mix.			
18. Placed medication label on bag (i.e., medication, dose, date, time, signature).			
Adding Medications to a Volume Administration Set Chamber			
19. Selected appropriate syringe and needle to prepare medicine.			
20. Used sterile technique while reconstituting and drawing up medicine. Recapped needle.			
21. Checked label for third time.			
22. Took medication to client and verified client's identity.			
23. Opened clamp between main IV bag and chamber and filled chamber with required amount of fluid (i.e., 50 to 100 ml.). Closed clamp.			
24. Cleaned injection site on chamber with alcohol swab.			
25. Inserted needle and injected medication into port.			
26. Removed needle and syringe and rotated chamber to mix.			
27. Ensured that IV was infusing at correct rate to deliver medication in appropriate amount of time.			
28. Placed medication label on bag (i.e., medicine, dose, date, time, signature).			
29. Flushed chamber and tubing with 10 to 20 ml. of fluid from IV bag after medication infused.			
30. Refilled chamber and continued infusion at ordered rate.			
Administering Medications with a Piggyback/Secondary Bag			
31. Selected appropriate syringe and needle to prepare medication.			
32. Used sterile technique while reconstituting and drawing up medication. Recapped needle.			
33. Checked label for third time.			

	S	U	COMMENTS
34. Obtained piggyback/secondary bag and discarded protective covering.			
35. Cleaned injection port and injected medication into bag through port of secondary set.			
36. Rotated bag to mix.			
37. Placed medication label on bag.			
38. Obtained a piggyback administration tubing set.			
39. Took to client and verified client identity.			
40. Uncapped spike on piggyback administration set and inserted it into admixture bag.			
41. Filled/flushed the tubing with admixture fluid and hung the piggyback on IV pole. Lowered the main IV (with hook provided) below the piggyback bag.			
42. Cleaned the appropriate injection port on main IV bag and inserted the needle from the piggyback set. Taped the connection.			
43. Regulated the infusion rate so that the medication would infuse in required amount time (i.e., 30 to 60 minutes).			
Administering Medication Through a Heparin or Saline Lock			
44. Selected appropriate syringe and needle to prepare medication.			
45. Used sterile technique while reconstituting and drawing up medication.			
46. Checked label for third time.			
47. Obtained appropriate bag of IV fluid and injected medication into it through injection port.			
48. Obtained IV administration tubing (unless already at bedside), spiked bag, flushed tubing and attached a sterile needle to end of tubing.			
49. Drew up 2 cc of saline into separate syringe and took to client along with medication.			
50. Verified client's identity.			

	S	U	COMMENTS
51. Cleaned injection port of heparin lock with alcohol swab and inserted needle from one saline filled syringe to check potency and flush heparin lock.			
52. Withdrew needle. Hung the bag with medication in it on IV pole and inserted the needle (on the tubing) into the injection port of the heparin lock.			
53. Released the clamp on the bag and regulated the flow rate to allow med to infuse over required time (i.e., 30 to 60 minutes).			
54. When infusion completed, flushed lock with 2 cc saline and instilled heparin if ordered.			
55. Remained with client for appropriate amount of time after giving med (i.e., check for side effects, allergic reaction, etc.).			
56. Disposed of equipment according to agency policy.			
57. Washed hands.			
58. Monitored infusion and assessed for effects of the medication.			
59. Appropriately documented the administration including assessment data and client response.			

Additional Comments:

_____

_____

_____

_____

_____

_____

_____

_____

_____

_____

_____

Name _____

Date _____

Instructor _____

Specific Skill Performed _____

Attempt Number _____

PASS _____   FAIL _____

PERFORMANCE CHECKLIST 19.1   ADMINISTERING AN INTRAVENOUS INFUSION

	S	U	COMMENTS
1. Checked physician's order and determined purpose of venipuncture.			
2. Explained procedure to client and positioned bed at comfortable working height.			
3. Washed hands.			
4. Gathered appropriate equipment, i.e., correct IV fluids, IV tubing or heparin lock, antiseptic pledget, correct needle.			
Preparing the Intravenous Solution			
5. Checked IV bag for leaks, expiration date, and color of fluids.			
6. Correctly calculated drip rate for infusion.			
7. Using sterile technique, connected tubing to bag and filled tubing with IV solution removing all air bubbles.			
8. Labeled IV bag and tubing correctly.			
Preparing to Insert an Intravenous Needle			
9. Assessed condition of veins and noted presence of bruises or hematomas.			
10. Closed the clamp and replaced protective cover over end of tubing.			
11. Positioned client so that vein is readily accessible.			
12. Cut or tore tape.			
13. Applied gloves.			
14. Shaved area where venipuncture is to be performed, if necessary.			
15. Placed moisture-proof pad under arm and applied tourniquet. Correctly scrubbed area with antiseptic pledget and allowed to dry.			
16. Removed protective cap from sterile needle, held needle in dominant hand and held vein taut with nondominant hand.			

	S	U	COMMENTS
17. Placed needle in line with vein at 15° to 45° angle, inserted needle with bevel up through skin into vein.			
18. If used over-the-needle catheter, advanced catheter into vein correctly and removed needle.			

Attaching the Intravenous Infusion

	S	U	COMMENTS
19. Removed protective cap and connected IV tubing to hub of catheter.			
20. Removed tourniquet and opened roller clamp to start infusion.			
21. Dressed IV site correctly and taped securely in place.			
22. Adjusted flow rate as ordered by physician.			
23. Labeled insertion site correctly.			

Final Activities

	S	U	COMMENTS
24. Disposed of supplies and equipment appropriately.			
25. Removed gloves and washed hands.			
26. Documented position and rate of IV, and response of client.			

Additional Comments:

_____

_____

_____

_____

_____

_____

_____

_____

_____

_____

_____

Name _____   Specific Skill Performed _____
Date _____   Attempt Number _____
Instructor _____   PASS _____   FAIL _____

PERFORMANCE CHECKLIST 19.2   **INSERTING A HEPARIN OR SALINE LOCK**

	S	U	COMMENTS
1. Ascertained if present IV can be converted or if new IV line is needed (see Performance Checklist 19.1).			
2. Washed hands and applied gloves.			
3. Explained procedure to client.			
4. Stopped IV infusion and disconnected tubing from catheter or needle.			
5. Immediately inserted adaptor into catheter or needle hub.			
6. If new IV catheter inserted, inserted end of intermittent adaptor into hub of catheter or needle.			
7. Taped the lock securely in place.			
8. Cleansed rubber diaphragm cap with alcohol swab and injected sterile saline and correct dose of heparin into lock.			
9. Dressed and labeled site correctly.			
10. Disposed of supplies and equipment appropriately.			
11. Removed gloves and washed hands.			
12. Documented insertion of lock and amount of heparin injected.			

Additional Comments:

_____

_____

_____

_____

_____

_____

Name _____   Specific Skill Performed _____
Date _____   Attempt Number _____
Instructor _____   PASS _____   FAIL _____

PERFORMANCE CHECKLIST 19.3   **CHANGING INTRAVENOUS TUBING AND AN IN-LINE FILTER**

	S	U	COMMENTS
1. Assessed need for changing tubing and filter.			
2. Explained procedure to client.			
3. Gathered appropriate equipment.			
4. Washed hands and applied gloves.			
5. Removed new tubing and filter from package without contaminating them.			
6. Removed the protective caps and connected the male end of the IV tubing to the female end of the filter.			
7. Closed IV clamp on old tubing and took IV bag off pole.			
8. Held IV bag upside-down while disconnecting tubing from bag.			
9. Taped drip chamber to IV pole without contaminating spike.			
10. Closed clamp on new tubing and inserted into upside-down IV bag.			
11. Hug bag on IV pole and filled tubing with IV fluid removing all air bubbles.			
12. Held filter upside-down to expel air as IV fluid goes through.			
13. Untaped old tubing from hub of IV needle, closed clamp, and stabilized needle or catheter while removing old tubing.			
14. Quickly attached end of new tubing to hub of needle or catheter without contaminating it.			
15. Opened the clamp and adjusted flow to ordered rate.			
16. Removed gloves and taped needle or catheter securely in place.			
17. Labeled tubing correctly.			
18. Disposed of equipment and old tubing appropriately.			
19. Assessed IV line for patency.			
20. Documented procedure correctly.			

Name _____

Date _____

Instructor _____

Specific Skill Performed _____

Attempt Number _____

PASS _____   FAIL _____

PERFORMANCE CHECKLIST 19.4   DISCONTINUING AN INTRAVENOUS INFUSION

1. Checked physician's order.			
2. Explained procedure to client.			
3. Washed hands and applied gloves.			
4. Closed clamp on IV tubing and carefully removed tape securing the IV.			
5. Held sterile gauze square over site as IV needle was gently removed.			
6. Immediately after removal of IV needle, applied firm pressure to gauze over site.			
7. After bleeding stopped, assessed site for signs of infection.			
8. Covered site with small bandage.			
9. Disposed of contaminated equipment properly.			
10. Removed gloves and washed hands.			
11. Documented removal of IV, amount of fluid in the IV bag, and condition of IV site.			

Additional Comments:

_____

_____

_____

_____

_____

_____

_____

_____

_____

Name _____   Specific Skill Performed _____
Date _____   Attempt Number _____
Instructor _____   PASS _____   FAIL _____

PERFORMANCE CHECKLIST 19.5   CHANGING THE GOWN OF A CLIENT WITH AN
INTRAVENOUS LINE

	S	U	COMMENTS
1. Assessed client's self-care abilities and mobility.			
2. Explained procedure to client.			
3. Washed hands and applied gloves.			
4. Obtained clean gown.			
5. Removed client's arms from sleeves of soiled gown.			
6. Placed clean gown over client or covered client with sheet or bath blanket.			
7. Removed IV bag from pole and slipped from front to back through armhole of soiled gown.			
8. If IV is infusing through a pump, clamped off tubing, turned off pump, and removed tubing from pump.			
9. Continuing to hold IV bag above client's arm, placed bag and tubing through sleeve of clean gown from back to front.			
10. Returned bag to IV pole and carefully slipped IV arm through sleeve of clean gown.			
11. Placed non-IV arm through sleeve of clean gown.			
12. Tied gown in back for client.			
13. Checked flow rate of IV and adjusted to correct rate if necessary. Reconnected to pump if necessary.			
14. Disposed of soiled gown appropriately.			
15. Ensured patency of IV and tubing and comfort of client.			

Additional Comments:

_____

_____

_____

_____

Name _____   Specific Skill Performed _____
Date _____   Attempt Number _____
Instructor _____   PASS _____   FAIL _____

PERFORMANCE CHECKLIST 19.6   **USING INFUSION DEVICES**

	S	U	COMMENTS
1. Checked physician's order for type and rate of IV solution.			
2. Washed hands.			
3. Gathered proper and clean equipment.			
4. Explained procedure to client.			
5. Placed a time line on bag of IV fluids.			
6. Inserted tubing spike correctly into bag of IV fluids using sterile technique.			
7. Filled the drip chamber 1/2 to 2/3 full for drop-calibrated infusion device or completely full for volume control device.			
8. Hung bag of IV fluids on IV pole attached to infusion device.			
9. Attached and threaded tubing through infusion device according to manufacturer's directions.			
10. Plugged infusion device into electrical outlet.			
11. Set the infusion rate or volume on pump.			
12. Inserted IV needle or catheter if necessary (see Performance Checklist 19.1). Attached tubing leading from the infusion device to the IV catheter.			
13. Opened tubing clamp completely.			
14. Turned the infusion device on using the power button.			
15. Checked to see that infusion device is delivering fluid correctly.			
16. Assessed IV site for signs of complications.			
17. Documented procedure correctly.			

Additional Comments:

_____

_____

_____

Name _____   Specific Skill Performed _____
Date _____   Attempt Number _____
Instructor _____   PASS _____   FAIL _____

PERFORMANCE CHECKLIST 19.7   **PROVIDING SITE CARE FOR A VASCULAR ACCESS DEVICE**

	S	U	COMMENTS
1. Checked whether procedure is to be sterile or clean.			
2. Gathered appropriate equipment.			
3. Explained procedure to client.			
4. Washed hands and applied gloves.			
5. Opened sterile supplies and placed them on the clean overbed table.			
6. Helped client assume a supine or semi-Fowler's position.			
7. Removed dressing on exit site of catheter and disposed of properly.			
8. Assessed site for signs of infection.			
9. Removed gloves and washed hands.			
10. Moistened sterile swabs with hydrogen peroxide.			
11. Cleansed skin around exit site in a circular motion from the center out.			
12. Held port of catheter in one hand while cleaning from exit site to port with alcohol swabs.			
13. Repeat procedure with povidone-iodine swabs.			
14. Applied small amount of povidone-iodine ointment to catheter exit site.			
15. Applied sterile occlusive dressing correctly.			
16. Labeled dressing correctly.			
17. Looped catheter loosely over the dressing and secured it with tape.			
18. Documented procedure correctly.			

Additional Comments:

_____

_____

PERFORMANCE CHECKLIST 20.1 CLEANSING A WOUND

	S	U	COMMENTS
1. Checked chart for physician's order/rationale for specific wound care and determined type of wound. Checked for allergies (i.e., antiseptics, etc.).			
2. Assessed client condition and size/location of the wound. Determined need for additional supplies.			
3. Obtained appropriate supplies and took to bedside.			
4. Explained procedure to client/family. Told client what to expect.			
5. Provided privacy, raised bed, lowered side rail and assisted client to comfortable position that allowed easy access to wound site.			
6. Exposed wound and draped client appropriately.			
7. Protected client's bed with waterproof pad/towel placed to absorb excess moisture.			
8. Prepared an easily accessible waterproof bag for disposal of soiled dressing/supplies.			
9. Put on clean gloves. Put on mask and other protective gear as needed.			
10. Used correct technique to remove soiled dressing and tape (i.e., supported skin proximal to tape and gently pulled tape toward wound). Loosened all around before lifting dressing off (underside away from client's face).			
11. Disposed of soiled dressing/tape in waterproof bag.			
12. Removed gloves (inside out) and placed in bag with dressing.			
13. Washed hands.			
14. Set up easily accessible sterile field and added sterile supplies. Did not contaminate field.			
15. Used proper technique to add cleaning solution to sterile basin. Did not wet sterile field.			
16. Put on sterile gloves.			

	S	U	COMMENTS

17. Used appropriate technique to clean wound.
   a. Used sterile forceps to pick up/saturate sterile 4 x 4 gauze.
   b. Cleaned wound one stroke at a time from cleanest area to least clean.
   c. Used a new gauze pad for each cleansing action.			

18. Discarded soiled gauze in waterproof bag.			
19. Rinsed wound in same manner using normal saline.			
20. Dried wound (same action) with dry pads.			
21. Applied dressing if appropriate (i.e., immediately post-op, ordered by physician, draining wound, etc.).			
22. Removed gloves (inside out) and discarded with soiled supplies. Disposed of bag according to agency policy.			
23. Returned client to position of comfort and lowered bed.			
24. Washed hands.			
25. Assessed client condition.			
26. Documented procedure including assessment data and client response.			

Additional Comments:

_____

_____

_____

_____

_____

_____

_____

_____

_____

_____

_____

Name _____   Specific Skill Performed _____
Date _____   Attempt Number _____
Instructor _____   PASS _____   FAIL _____

PERFORMANCE CHECKLIST 20.2   IRRIGATING AND PACKING A WOUND

	S	U	COMMENTS
1. Checked client's chart for physician's order/rationale, type of wound, prior wound assessment data, and to determine irrigation solution.			
2. Assessed client's condition (i.e., comfort level) and inquired about prior wound irrigations. Explained procedure/purpose to client/family and told them what to expect.			
3. Administered analgesic if indicated.			
4. Gathered supplies while analgesic is becoming effective.			
5. Provided privacy, raised bed, lowered side rail and positioned client so that wound would be easily accessible. Closed doors, windows, and curtains in client's room.			
6. Washed hands.			
7. Exposed wound and draped client appropriately.			
8. Protected client's bed with waterproof pad. Placed a collecting basin at bottom of wound.			
9. Prepared an easily accessible waterproof bag for disposal of soiled supplies.			
10. Prepared sterile field and added necessary supplies for irrigating and packing wound.			
11. Put on gloves, goggles, gown, and other protective gear as needed.			
12. Used appropriate technique to remove soiled dressing and tape. Disposed of dressing in waterproof bag.			
13. Removed wound packing, if present, and placed in bag with soiled dressing.			
14. Assessed wound (i.e., depth, width, general appearance, redness, tenderness, exudate, necrotic tissue, granulation tissue, odor, etc.).			
15. Removed soiled exam gloves and discarded.			
16. Washed hands.			

	S	U	COMMENTS
Irrigating the Wound			
17. Put on sterile gloves.			

18. Withdrew 30 ml. of irrigant into syringe and irrigated wound:
  a. Held blunt needle tip 1 to 2" above wound.
  b. Flushed wound from top to bottom using gentle pressure.			

19. Used sterile 4 x 4 gauze pads to dry inside of wound (i.e., gently placed 4 x 4s inside wound to absorb fluid) and another one to dry skin around the wound. Did not touch wound with gloves.			
Packing the Wound			
20. Held forceps in dominant hand and packing material (i.e., gauze) in non-dominant hand. Used forceps to guide the gauze loosely into wound. Completely packed the wound.			

21. Finished dressing the wound:
  a. Placed sterile gauze pads on top of packing.
  b. Placed sterile abdominal pads over gauze pads.
  c. Secured dressing with tape or Montgomery straps (see Performance Checklist 20.4).			

22. Removed waterproof pad and assisted client to position of comfort. Lowered bed to lowest position.			
23. Disposed of soiled dressing and supplies according to agency policy.			
24. Removed gloves and washed hands.			
25. Documented the procedure including assessment data and client response.			

Additional Comments:

_____

_____

_____

_____

_____

_____

Name _____   Specific Skill Performed _____
Date _____   Attempt Number _____
Instructor _____   PASS _____   FAIL _____

PERFORMANCE CHECKLIST 20.3   APPLYING A DRY STERILE DRESSING

	S	U	COMMENTS
1. Checked client's chart for physician's order/rationale, type of wound, prior wound assessment data, and presence of drain.			
2. Assessed client's condition (i.e., comfort level) and inquired about prior dressing changes. Explained procedure/purpose to client/family and told them what to expect.			
3. Administered analgesic if indicated.			
4. Gathered supplies while analgesic is becoming effective.			
5. Provided privacy, raised bed, lowered side rail and positioned client so that wound would be easily accessible. Closed doors, windows, and curtains in client's room.			
6. Washed hands.			
7. Exposed wound and draped client appropriately.			
8. Protected client's bed with waterproof pad.			
9. Prepared an easily accessible waterproof bag for disposal of soiled supplies.			
10. Prepared sterile field and added necessary supplies.			
11. Put on gloves, goggles, gown, and other protective gear as needed.			
12. Used appropriate technique to remove soiled dressing and tape. Disposed of dressing in waterproof bag.			
13. Assessed wound (i.e., depth, width, general appearance, redness, tenderness, exudate, necrotic tissue, granulation tissue, odor, etc.).			
14. Removed soiled exam gloves and discarded.			
15. Washed hands.			
16. Put on sterile gloves.			
17. Cleaned wound as needed (see Performance Checklist 20.1).			

	S	U	COMMENTS
18. Folded 4 x 4 gauze pad in half and applied it lengthwise on wound.			
19. Continued to apply gauze 4 x 4s until wound completely covered. Anticipated area where most drainage would occur and added extra pads over area.			
20. If penrose drain present, used pre-cut drain sponge (if available) around drain and reinforced with additional 4 x 4s on top.			
21. Placed sterile abdominal pad over 4 x 4s.			
22. Applied tape to hold dressing in place or secured with Montgomery straps if appropriate (see Performance Checklist 20.4).			
23. Assisted client to position of comfort and lowered bed.			
24. Disposed of soiled dressing and supplies according to agency policy.			
25. Removed gloves and washed hands.			
26. Documented the procedure including assessment data and client response.			

Additional Comments:

_____

_____

_____

_____

_____

_____

_____

_____

_____

_____

_____

_____

Name _____   Specific Skill Performed _____
Date _____   Attempt Number _____
Instructor _____   PASS _____   FAIL _____

PERFORMANCE CHECKLIST 20.4   USING MONTGOMERY STRAPS

	S	U	COMMENTS
1. Assessed wound and determined if multiple dressing changes anticipated.			
2. Gathered supplies and took to client's bedside.			
3. Explained procedure/purpose to client/family.			
4. Provided privacy, raised bed and assisted client to appropriate position.			
5. Draped client and exposed wound.			

6. Prepared Montgomery straps (or opened commercial ones) and placed them for easy accessibility.
  a. Correctly estimated length of tape needed for client's wound (i.e., 2" attachment to skin and sufficient non-adherent surface to overlay wound).
  b. Cut small hole in end of non-adherent tab(s).			

7. Put on gloves and removed soiled dressing.			
8. Used sterile technique to administer wound care and re-dress wound as ordered/per protocol/agency guidelines (see Performance Checklists 20.1, 20.2, and 20.3).			
9. Applied Montgomery straps to client's skin with the non-adherent tabs facing toward the suture line. Placed straps so that opposing tabs did not completely meet or overlap at suture line.			
10. Used gauze (or umbilical tape) to lace or tie the straps together over the dressing. Secured the ties with a loose knot or bow tie.			
11. Assisted client to position of comfort and lowered the bed.			
12. Disposed of soiled equipment/supplies (if not already done).			
13. Washed hands.			
14. Documented the dressing change including assessment data, wound care, use of Montgomery straps, and client response.			

PERFORMANCE CHECKLIST 20.5   APPLYING A WET-TO-DRY DRESSING

		S	U	COMMENTS
1.	Checked client's chart for physician's order/rationale and type of solution to be used for wet dressing.			
2.	Assessed client's condition (i.e., comfort level) and explained procedure to client/family.			
3.	Assessed wound to determine if extra supplies needed.			
4.	Administered analgesic if indicated.			
5.	Provided privacy, raised bed, lowered side rail, and positioned client so that wound would be easily accessible. Closed doors, windows, and curtains in client's room.			
6.	Washed hands.			
7.	Exposed wound and draped client appropriately.			
8.	Protected client bed with a waterproof pad.			
9.	Prepared an easily accessible waterproof bag for disposal of soiled supplies.			
10.	Put on clean gloves (and other protective gear if needed).			
11.	Used appropriate technique to remove and dispose of soiled dressing. Was careful not to moisten dressing. Lifted dressing straight up (i.e., 90^0 angle to wound) and held inside away from client's face. Removed wound packing.			
12.	Assessed wound (i.e., depth, width, general appearance, redness, tenderness, exudate, necrotic tissue, granulation tissue, odor, etc.).			
13.	Removed soiled gloves and discarded.			
14.	Washed hands.			
15.	Set up sterile field and added necessary supplies (including prescribed solution).			
16.	Put on sterile gloves.			

	S	U	COMMENTS
17. Picked up 4 x 4 gauze (soaked with prescribed solution in basin), squeezed it to remove excess liquid, and opened it completely.			
18. Held gauze in non-dominant hand and used forceps (in dominant hand) to guide the gauze into client's wound until all inner surfaces are covered.			
19. Placed a dry 4 x 4 gauze over the moistened dressing.			
20. Placed an abdominal pad over the wound and dressing.			
21. Secured the dressing with tape or with Montgomery straps (see Performance Checklist 20.4). Was careful not to make the dressing occlusive.			
22. Positioned client for comfort, raised side rail and lowered bed.			
23. Disposed of soiled dressing and supplies according to agency policy.			
24. Removed gloves and washed hands.			
25. Documented the procedure including assessment data and client response.			

Additional Comments:

_____

_____

_____

_____

_____

_____

_____

_____

_____

_____

_____

Name _____   Specific Skill Performed _____

Date _____   Attempt Number _____

Instructor _____   PASS _____   FAIL _____

PERFORMANCE CHECKLIST 20.6 APPLYING A TRANSPARENT DRESSING

	S	U	COMMENTS
1. Checked client's chart for prior wound assessment data.			
2. Assessed client's condition/wound condition and determined if additional supplies needed.			
3. Explained procedure/purpose to client/family.			
4. Provided privacy, raised bed, lowered side rail, and positioned client so that wound would be easily accessible.			
5. Exposed wound. Draped client if appropriate and protected bed if needed.			
6. Put on clean gloves.			
7. Used appropriate technique to remove old dressing (i.e., held skin taut, lifted edge of dressing, and pulled it off in direction of hair growth).			
8. Discarded dressing appropriately.			
9. Assessed the wound (i.e., approximation of edges, edema, redness, warmth, drainage, etc.).			
10. Provided wound care as ordered.			
11. Removed gloves and discarded.			
12. Washed hands.			
13. Opened new transparent dressing package.			
14. Put on gloves (sterile if appropriate).			
15. Separated approximately 1" of the backing on the transparent dressing and placed the dressing directly over the area to be covered.			
16. Held the dressing in place with one hand while continuing to remove the backing and placing the dressing with the other. Slowly smoothed and applied the dressing to the site.			
17. Reinforced the edges of the dressing with tape (i.e., picture frame) if necessary.			

	S	U	COMMENTS
18. Dated, timed, and initialed the new dressing.			
19. Positioned client for comfort, raised rail, and lowered bed.			
20. Removed gloves and washed hands.			
21. Documented the dressing change including assessment data and client response.			

Additional Comments:

_____

_____

_____

_____

_____

_____

_____

_____

_____

_____

_____

_____

_____

_____

_____

_____

_____

Name _____   Specific Skill Performed _____

Date _____   Attempt Number _____

Instructor _____   PASS _____   FAIL _____

PERFORMANCE CHECKLIST 20.7   MANAGING WOUND DRAINS AND WOUND SUCTION DEVICES

	S	U	COMMENTS
Cleaning and Dressing a Drain Site and Shortening a Penrose Drain			
Cleaning and Dressing a Drain Site			
1. Checked client's chart for physician's order regarding dressing change and shortening of Penrose drain.			
2. Obtained a suture removal kit and sterile safety pin in addition to supplies needed to clean/dress client's wound.			
3. Followed steps in Performance Checklist 20.1 to clean incision site. Maintained sterile technique throughout procedure.			
4. Lifted up drain with hemostat (non-dominant hand) and with forceps (in dominant hand), cleaned drain site with saline-soaked gauze pad (or cotton-tipped applicator). Cleaned in a circular pattern from inner to outer area around drain.			
Shortening the Penrose Drain			
5. Released suture holding the drain in place (with suture removal kit).			
6. Grasped Penrose drain with forceps (across entire width, close to client's skin) and pulled drain out for the ordered number of inches.			
7. Inserted a sterile safety pin through the drain as close to client's skin as possible.			
8. Cut off excess drain with sterile scissors 2" from skin and discarded cut-off portion with soiled dressing.			
9. Reapplied dressing to the wound and drain site (see Performance Checklist 20.5).			
10. Documented the procedure including assessment data, how much drain was shortened, client response, etc.			

	S	U	COMMENTS
Emptying a Closed Wound Drainage System and Reestablishing Suction			
11. Put on clean gloves.			
12. Opened drain plug, inverted the drainage receptacle and drained the contents into a graduated collection container.			
Reestablishing Suction in a Hemovac			
13. Placed Hemovac on a firm, flat surface, compressed the evacuation receptacle and closed the drain plug while maintaining compression on the device.			
Reestablishing Suction in a Jackson-Pratt			
14. Held Jackson-Pratt bulb in hand, compressed the evacuation receptacle and closed the drain plug while maintaining compression on the bulb.			
15. Removed gloves and washed hands.			
16. Documented the procedure.			

Additional Comments:

_____

_____

_____

_____

_____

_____

_____

_____

_____

_____

_____

PERFORMANCE CHECKLIST 20.8   **REMOVING SUTURES**

	S	U	COMMENTS
1. Checked client's chart for physician's order regarding suture removal.			
2. Obtained suture removal kit and other needed supplies.			
3. Explained procedure/purpose to client/family.			
4. Provided privacy, raised bed, lowered rail, and assisted client to position that provides easy access and visibility of suture line. Closed windows, doors, and curtains.			
5. Draped client appropriately and exposed wound.			
6. Assessed wound to determine if edges are well-approximated and healing has occurred.			
7. Put on clean gloves, removed dressing, and placed it in a disposable bag.			
8. Removed gloves and washed hands.			
9. Opened suture removal kit/other supplies and placed them for easy accessibility.			
10. Put on sterile gloves and provided wound care (i.e., cleaned wound with pads soaked in saline or antiseptic swabs).			
11. **Removal of Interrupted Suture:** Grasped suture near knot with forceps (non-dominant hand). Slipped curbed edge of scissors under suture and cut it (dominant hand). Pulled it with forceps to remove.			
12. **Removal of Continuous Suture:** Cut both the first and second suture before removing them.			
13. Removed every other suture and reassessed the suture line.			
14. Discarded sutures into gauze square and placed it into bag with soiled dressing.			
15. Applied adhesive strips or butterfly tape adhesive strips across suture line to secure edges if appropriate.			
16. Discarded soiled equipment.			

	S	U	COMMENTS
17. Assisted client to position of comfort and lowered bed.			
18. Removed gloves and washed hands.			
19. Documented the procedure including assessment data (i.e., appearance of suture line, etc.) and client response.			

Additional Comments:

_____

_____

_____

_____

_____

_____

_____

_____

_____

_____

_____

_____

_____

_____

_____

_____

_____

_____

Name _____   Specific Skill Performed _____

Date _____   Attempt Number _____

Instructor _____   PASS _____   FAIL _____

PERFORMANCE CHECKLIST 20.9 REMOVING STAPLES

	S	U	COMMENTS
1. Checked client's chart for physician's order regarding staple removal.			
2. Obtained staple extractor and other needed supplies.			
3. Explained procedure/purpose to client/family.			
4. Provided privacy, raised bed, lowered rail, and assisted client to position that provides easy access and visibility of suture line. Closed windows, doors, and curtains.			
5. Draped client appropriately and exposed wound.			
6. Assessed wound to determine if edges are well approximated and healing has occurred.			
7. Put on clean gloves, removed dressing and placed it in a disposable bag.			
8. Removed gloves and washed hands.			
9. Opened staple extractor/other supplies and placed them for easy accessibility.			
10. Put on sterile gloves and provided wound care (i.e., cleaned wound with pads soaked in saline or antiseptic swabs).			
11. Placed lower edge of staple extractor under first staple.			
12. Pressed the handles of the staple extractor together and lifted the staple out of the client's skin.			
13. Moved the staple over to a gauze pad while the handles were still pressed together, then released the handles.			
14. Continued the process, and removed every other staple.			
15. Reassessed the suture line to ensure that edges were well approximated.			
16. Removed all staples if suture line appeared well-healed.			
17. Applied adhesive strips or butterfly tape adhesive strips across suture line if appropriate.			

	S	U	COMMENTS
18. Discarded soiled equipment.			
19. Assisted client to position of comfort and lowered bed.			
20. Removed gloves and washed hands.			
21. Documented the procedure including assessment data and client response.			

Additional Comments:

_____

_____

_____

_____

_____

_____

_____

_____

_____

_____

_____

_____

_____

_____

_____

_____

_____

Name _____

Date _____

Instructor _____

Specific Skill Performed _____

Attempt Number _____

PASS _____   FAIL _____

PERFORMANCE CHECKLIST 20.10 PROVIDING UMBILICAL CORD CARE FOR AN INFANT

	S	U	COMMENTS
Initial Cord Care			
1. Checked agency policy regarding cord care.			
2. Assessed condition of cord (i.e., presence of arteries, veins, color, etc.) when infant arrived in nursery.			
3. Obtained supplies and put on gloves.			
4. Opened container of triple-dye solution.			
5. Gently raised stump upwards off baby's abdomen.			
6. Used a swab, soaked with triple-dye solution, to coat the stump. Began at clamp, proceeded to base of stump and then, in a circular motion, swabbed from stump outwards for 1".			
7. Removed gloves and washed hands.			
8. Assessed parents' knowledge/ability to care for cord following discharge. Discussed procedure with them.			
9. Documented the procedure including assessment data, solution used, and any teaching/learning activities.			
Subsequent Cord Care			
10. Put on gloves.			
11. At each diaper change, lifted umbilical stump off abdomen and swabbed it with cotton ball soaked with alcohol.			
12. At discharge, (or 2 days old), removed the umbilical clamp.			
13. Removed gloves and washed hands.			
14. Documented the procedure including assessment data.			

Additional Comments:

_____

_____

Name _____   Specific Skill Performed _____
Date _____   Attempt Number _____
Instructor _____   PASS _____   FAIL _____

PERFORMANCE CHECKLIST 20.11 **PROVIDING CIRCUMCISION CARE**

	S	U	COMMENTS
1. Checked client's chart for physician's order/rationale for the procedure.			
2. Ensured that consent form was signed by parents.			
3. Discussed procedure with parents. Explained what to expect during and after the circumcision.			
4. Gathered equipment/supplies and placed them for easy accessibility.			
5. Removed infant's diaper.			
6. Restrained infant on circumcision board.			
7. Administered analgesic as ordered by physician.			
8. Assessed infant's response during circumcision (i.e., pain).			
9. Attempted to distract/soothe infant by stroking his forehead and talking calmly to him.			
10. After procedure completed, put on sterile gloves and applied petroleum jelly gauze to site.			
11. Assessed the circumcision site for bleeding.			
12. Placed infant on his side with diaper loosely attached.			
13. Removed gloves and washed hands.			
14. Observed infant void and assessed for adequacy of stream, amount voided, and presence of blood.			
15. Taught parents how to assess for evidence of infection and to report it immediately.			
16. If Plastibell was used, told parents that it would fall off in 3 to 4 days.			
17. Documented the procedure including assessment data (i.e., amount of bleeding, edema and voiding pattern, client response, and any teaching/learning activities).			

Name _____   Specific Skill Performed _____
Date _____   Attempt Number _____
Instructor _____   PASS _____   FAIL _____

PERFORMANCE CHECKLIST 20.12 APPLYING BANDAGE WRAPS

	S	U	COMMENTS
1. Checked client's chart to determine area to be bandaged, type of bandage to be applied, and rationale for bandage.			
2. Discussed procedure/purpose with client/family.			
3. Assessed area to be bandaged (i.e., broken areas, redness, swelling) and determined amount of supplies needed.			
4. Gathered supplies and took to client.			
5. Provided privacy and assisted client to position that allowed for easy access of area to be bandaged.			
6. Applied bandage.			
Applying an Arm Sling			
7. Properly placed sling across client's chest under the affected arm (i.e., apex extending beyond elbow, upper point of triangle across clavicle on unaffected side and extending behind and around neck).			
8. Positioned arm appropriately (80° or lower), brought bottom half of sling up over arm and tied/fastened it to portion of sling around neck (i.e., square knot or safety pin).			
9. Folded the remaining cloth (at elbow) and secured it with a safety pin.			
10. Reassessed angle of arm, inspected clavicle, and padded knot if needed.			
Applying a Bandage Using Circular Turns			
11. With dominant hand, placed rolls of gauze (flat surface down) on top of surface to be bandaged.			
12. Unrolled the gauze. Overlapped and circled the area (i.e., digit or arm) two times.			
13. Cut the gauze with scissors, folded the ends under and secured the end of the gauze with tape.			

	S	U	COMMENTS

Applying a Bandage Using Spiral Turns

	S	U	COMMENTS
14. Anchored the bandage at the distal end of part to be bandaged with two circular turns.			
15. Applied the bandage from the distal end to the proximal border by overlapping the previous turn 1/2 to 3/4 the width of the bandage.			
16. Cut the end of the bandage with scissors, folded it under, and secured it with tape.			

Applying a Bandage Using Spiral Reverse Turns

	S	U	COMMENTS
17. Anchored the bandage at the distal end with two circular turns.			
18. Used appropriate technique to apply the bandage from the distal border to the proximal border (i.e., 30° angle advancement of bandage on anterior surface, then folded back/reversed to form inverted "V" to be wrapped around posterior aspect of part and repeated until completely covered).			
19. Completed bandaging with two circular turns.			
20. Cut bandage and secured with tape.			

Applying a Bandage Using a Figure-of-Eight Turn

	S	U	COMMENTS
21. Anchored bandage at the distal end with two circular turns.			
22. Advanced the bandage above the joint, circled it around the back and brought it down to cross over the front of the joint.			
23. Continued to wrap the bandage above and below the joint (figure-of-eight turns) until the joint was completely wrapped.			
24. Completed bandage with two circular turns.			
25. Cut bandage and secured with tape.			

Applying a Bandage Using Recurrent Turns

	S	U	COMMENTS
26. Anchored the bandage with two circular turns around the proximal area (i.e., limb stump or head).			

	S	U	COMMENTS
27. Made a reverse turn in center front, advanced gauze toward back and reversed the gauze in center back. Brought the gauze to center front and again reversed it.			
28. Continued the reverse turns until the entire body part was covered.			
29. Completed the bandaging with two circular turns.			
30. Cut the bandage and secured it with tape.			
31. Documented the procedure including assessment data (i.e., skin integrity, color, temperature, levels of comfort, etc.) and client response.			

Additional Comments:

_____

_____

_____

_____

_____

_____

_____

_____

_____

_____

_____

_____

_____

_____

_____

_____

_____

PERFORMANCE CHECKLIST 20.13 APPLYING BINDERS

		S	U	COMMENTS
1.	Checked client's chart to determine area to be bound and type of/rationale for binder.			
2.	Discussed procedure/purpose with client/family.			
3.	Assessed area to be bound (i.e., broken areas, redness, swelling) and determined size binder needed (i.e., small, large, extra large, etc.).			
4.	Obtained binder and took to client.			
5.	Provided privacy, raised bed, lowered side rail, and assisted client to supine position.			
6.	Applied binder.			
Applying a Breast Binder				
7.	Removed gown and draped client appropriately.			
8.	If a rectangular muslin cloth was used: a. Placed the cloth behind the client's back. b. Brought the binder edges up around the client's anterior chest while the client inhaled deeply. c. Overlapped the edges of the binder and pinned them together appropriately.			
9.	If a vest-style binder was used: a. Put the vest on the client and followed b and c above for closing and fastening the edges.			
Applying Straight and Scultetus Abdominal Binders				
10.	Ensured that opposite side rail was up and had client roll onto his/her side facing the raised side rail.			
11.	Fan-folded half of the binder lengthwise, placed it under client (between lower rib cage and symphysis pubis), raised remaining side rail and had client roll back onto binder and onto other side.			

	S	U	COMMENTS
12. Pulled/straightened the fan-folded portion of the binder beneath client and had client roll back to supine position with head and knees elevated slightly.			
Applying a Straight Binder			
13. Pulled the sides of the binder to meet together in the middle (vertically) and fastened them together (i.e., velcro or safety pins).			
Applying a Scultetus Binder			
14. Appropriately placed and overlapped each pair of tails (starting at left bottom) until all were secured in the middle. Maintained adequate tension on tails when overlapping them and secured top set with a safety pin.			
Applying T-Binders and Double T-Binders			
15. Assisted client to bend his/her knees and slightly raise buttocks.			
16. Properly placed the binder under the client (i.e., horizontal bands under waist, vertical band(s) under gluteal folds).			
17. Overlapped horizontal band around waist (above iliac crest) and secured with a safety pin.			
Securing a T-Binder			
18. Brought bottom portion of T-binder (vertical band) up between client's legs, over perineum, and under the waistband. Folded the flap over and secured with a safety pin.			
Securing a Double T-Binders			
19. Brought bottom portions of T-binder (vertical bands) up between client's legs, over scrotal and perineal area, and to either side of penis. Folded flaps over and secured them with safety pins.			
20. Assisted client to position of comfort and lowered bed.			
21. Documented the procedure including assessment data and client response.			

Name _____   Specific Skill Performed _____
Date _____   Attempt Number _____
Instructor _____   PASS _____   FAIL _____

PERFORMANCE CHECKLIST 20.14 **APPLYING A SPLINT**

	S	U	COMMENTS
1. Checked client's chart to determine area to be splinted, type of splint required and rationale for the use of splint.			
2. Explained procedure/purpose to client/family.			
3. Assessed area to be splinted (i.e., color, moisture, swelling/edema, pulses, capillary refill, intactness of skin, pain, numbness, etc.). Assessed circulation distal to area.			
4. Selected proper splint (i.e., size, shape) to immobilize the area.			
5. Applied the splint appropriately to support the area and inhibit movement.			
6. Assessed for circulation distal to splint.			
7. Washed hands.			
8. Documented the procedure including assessment data and client response.			
9. Reassessed splinted area periodically for distal circulation, effectiveness of immobilization, and client level of comfort.			

Additional Comments:

_____

_____

_____

_____

_____

_____

_____

_____

_____

Name _____   Specific Skill Performed _____

Date _____   Attempt Number _____

Instructor _____   PASS _____   FAIL _____

PERFORMANCE CHECKLIST 20.15 DRESSING AN AMPUTATED LIMB

	S	U	COMMENTS
1. Checked client's chart to determine date of surgery, surgical procedure, and relevant physician's orders.			
2. Explained procedure/purpose to client/family. Discussed client's preference regarding type of bandaging techniques if appropriate.			
3. Obtained supplies and took to client's room.			
4. Provided privacy, raised bed, lowered rail, and assisted client to supine position. Closed windows, doors, and curtains if suture line not healed. Draped client appropriately.			
5. Prepared a disposal bag, put on clean gloves, removed the old dressing, and discarded it in bag.			
6. Assessed the stump for size and stage of healing.			
7. Removed gloves and washed hands.			
8. Referred/followed Performance Checklist 20.1 to clean suture line, if needed (or followed agency policy).			
9. Placed unfolded 4 x 4 gauze pads over suture line of amputated limb. Removed and discarded gloves.			
10. Assisted client to semi-Fowler's position in bed (or sitting position on side of bed).			
11. Held elastic wrap in dominant hand (flat side down, roll facing upwards) and applied bandage.			
Figure-of-Eight Dressing for Above-the-Knee Amputations			
12. Anchored bandage with circular turns around the waist.			
13. Began at front of thigh and wrapped the bandage downward (at oblique angle) to inner aspect of stump.			
14. Wrapped the bandage around the medial and lateral aspects of stump, then around to the front of the stump, and circled bandage up around client's waist forming a figure-of-eight.			
15. Continued wrapping/overlapping the previous figure-of-eight turns until stump was covered.			

	S	U	COMMENTS
16. Anchored the bandage with tape, or metal clips provided with the elastic wrap.			
Recurrent Bandage for Above or Below-the-Knee Residual Limb or Amputation Below-the-Elbow			
17. Anchored bandage at proximal end of stump with two circular turns.			
18. Covered stump with recurrent turns (see Performance Checklist 20.12).			
19. Finished bandage with two circular turns at proximal end and secured bandage with tape or metal clips.			
Figure-of-Eight Bandage of Above-the-Elbow Residual Limb			
20. Anchored bandage with two circular turns and covered the end of the amputated limb with two recurrent turns.			
21. Used figure-of-eight turns to wrap the stump and around the client's back and shoulders.			
22. Secured the bandage with tape or metal clips.			
Spiral Bandage of Amputated Limb			
23. Covered distal end of stump with recurrent turns.			
24. Covered rest of stump (distal to proximal) with spiral turns.			
25. Anchored bandage around client's waist and secured it with tape or metal clips.			
After Bandaging Stump			
26. Assessed client's level of comfort and mobility of proximal joints. Assisted client to position of comfort and lowered bed.			
27. Disposed of soiled equipment/supplies.			
28. Documented the procedure including assessment data and client response.			

Name _____   Specific Skill Performed _____
Date _____   Attempt Number _____
Instructor _____   PASS _____   FAIL _____

PERFORMANCE CHECKLIST 20.16 **APPLYING A PRESSURE DRESSING**

	S	U	COMMENTS
Managing Sudden, Unexpected Bleeding *First Nurse*			
1. Quickly assessed site of hemorrhage and called for assistance.			
2. Applied direct pressure to hemorrhage site.			
3. Elevated extremity if appropriate.			
Second Nurse			
4. Gathered supplies (i.e., sterile compresses, tourniquet, etc.).			
5. Put on sterile gloves and quickly applied sterile compresses to hemorrhage site (as first nurse temporarily lifted fingers from site). Had first nurse reapply pressure immediately.			
Controlling and Preventing Bleeding			
6. Applied gauze around site completely covering dressing and wound. Had first nurse lift fingers for gauze placement and reapply pressure as quickly as possible between each layer.			
7. Prepared strips of tape (adequate in length and number) to completely cover the dressing and hemorrhage site.			
8. Applied overlapping strips of tape to form occlusive dressing. Snugly wrapped the site if elastic bandage used.			
9. Removed gloves and washed hands.			
10. Assessed client's condition (i.e., B/P, pulse, pulses distal to hemorrhage/bleeding site, extremity color/warmth/sensation).			

11. If hemorrhage sudden or unexpected:
   a. Notified MD and obtained orders.
   b. Started IV if ordered.
   c. Continued to monitor VS q 15 minutes until stable for 1°.			

12. Documented the intervention and follow-up actions including assessment data and client response.			

Name _____   Specific Skill Performed _____
Date _____   Attempt Number _____
Instructor _____   PASS _____   FAIL _____

PERFORMANCE CHECKLIST 20.17 **APPLYING A HYDROCOLLOID DRESSING**

	S	U	COMMENTS
1. Assessed dressing and determined need for dressing change.			
2. Checked client's chart for physician's order/rationale regarding dressing change.			
3. Obtained appropriate supplies for dressing change and wound care including correctly sized hydrocolloid dressing.			
4. Explained procedure/purpose to client/family.			
5. Provided privacy, raised bed, lowered side rail, and assisted client to position that allowed easy access to wound. Pulled curtains and closed doors and windows.			
6. Exposed wound and draped client. Protected bed with waterproof pad.			
7. Washed hands, put on clean gloves, and removed old dressing. Appropriately loosened the dressing on all sides and lifted it carefully.			
8. Discarded old dressing and gloves in waterproof, disposable bag.			
9. Washed hands.			
10. Used sterile technique to open/prepare/add supplies to sterile field (i.e., irrigation set, basin with saline, 4 x 4s, etc.). Peeled back corner of backing paper on granule packet and placed it for easy access.			
11. Put on sterile gloves.			
12. Irrigated wound (see Performance Checklist 20.2) as ordered (i.e., isotonic saline in 30 ml. syringe with 19-gauge blunt-tipped needle at 8 PSI pressure).			
13. Dried skin around wound with sterile 4 x 4 gauze pad.			
14. Assessed the clean wound (i.e., erythemas, odor, drainage, necrotic tissue, change in size or depth, etc.).			
15. Applied granules or paste if ordered. Did not fill wound higher than skin level.			

	S	U	COMMENTS
16. Peeled back the cover of the hydrocolloid dressing and discarded it. Used sterile scissors to cut the dressing into desired shape if needed.			
17. Appropriately applied the hydrocolloid dressing (i.e., directly onto wound, rolled into place from one side to other, smoothed edges, etc.). Did not stretch dressing.			
18. Removed gloves and discarded them.			
19. Taped the edges of the dressing in place (i.e., picture frame).			
20. Assisted client to position of comfort and lowered bed.			
21. Disposed of soiled dressing/equipment according to agency policy.			
22. Washed hands.			
23. Documented the procedure including assessment data and client response.			

Additional Comments:

_____

_____

_____

_____

_____

_____

_____

_____

_____

_____

_____

_____

_____

Name _____

Date _____

Instructor _____

Specific Skill Performed _____

Attempt Number _____

PASS _____   FAIL _____

PERFORMANCE CHECKLIST 21.1 POSTMORTEM CARE

	S	U	COMMENTS
1. Escorted family to private area where they were informed of client's death (i.e., by physician).			
2. Informed family that after a few minutes of preparation time, they might view the body.			
3. Inquired if family desired a religious person to be present (i.e., chaplain, priest, minister, etc.).			
4. Checked chart to determine if isolation precautions were necessary (i.e., presence of an infectious disease).			
5. Arranged for client's roommate/family to leave the room.			
6. Gathered appropriate equipment/supplies (including shroud kit) and brought to bedside.			
7. Washed hands and put on gloves.			
8. Checked arm band to identify client. Removed arm band.			
9. Placed client in supine position, arms at sides with palms down.			
10. Placed small pillow or folded towel under client's head.			
11. Gently closed eyes and held them in place for a few moments.			

12. Provided grooming/hygiene to client's head:
   a. Washed face.
   b. Combed hair and removed pins and clips.
   c. Inserted dentures. Placed rolled towel under chin.			

13. Provided grooming/hygiene to client's body:
   a. Disconnected all bags, bottles, and collection devices.
   b. Removed all tubes unless autopsy anticipated.
   c. Washed soiled body parts.
   d. Placed absorbent pad under buttocks.
   e. Attached ID tag to great toe or ankle.
   f. Put clean gown on body and covered with a clean sheet or blanket. Turned down cover so that head was exposed.			

14. Collected clothing/non-valuables and placed in bag to return to family.			

	S	U	COMMENTS
15. Collected valuables (including jewelry) and checked the valuable list to ascertain if all items present. Returned to next of kin and obtained signature. Taped wedding ring to finger at family request.			
16. Straightened room, softened the light and provided chairs for family.			
17. Obtained aromatic spirits of ammonia.			
18. Escorted family to bedside. Stayed with family a few minutes then gave them private time with deceased.			

19. After family departed, completed postmortem care:
  a. Exposed body and attached ID tag (from shroud kit) to great toe or ankle
  b. Wrapped ankles with pads and tied them together with gauze.
  c. Placed body in body bag or wrapped in shroud. If head was shaved, included client's hair.
  d. Attached ID tag to outside of bag.			

20. Cleared hallways and closed doors to other client's rooms.			
21. Obtained stretcher and took client to morgue.			
22. Removed gloves and washed hands.			
23. Documented procedure. Included time of death, events surrounding death, family notification, postmortem care given, disposition of clothing and valuables, permits obtained and time body was taken to morgue.			

Additional Comments:

_____

_____

_____

_____

_____

_____

_____

_____

_____

PERFORMANCE CHECKLIST A.1   TAKING A HEALTH HISTORY

	S	U	COMMENTS
1. Considered communication principles while conducting the interview.			
2. Provided for client privacy and confidentiality.			
3. Noticed verbal and nonverbal cues and assessed reliability.			
4. Obtained chief complaint which was specific and accurately described.			
5. History of present illness was described according to the 7 variables of symptomology.			
6. Obtained past medical history of previous illness, health promotion activities, allergies, and current medications and treatments.			
7. Assessed family history related to present illnesses and future health risks.			
8. Obtained information about personal and social history pertinent to health care.			
9. Obtained a review of systems in a systematic fashion gathering more information when necessary.			
10. Recorded health history correctly and accurately.			

Additional Comments:

_____

_____

_____

_____

_____

_____

_____

_____

_____

_____

Name _____ Specific Skill Performed _____

Date _____ Attempt Number _____

Instructor _____ PASS _____ FAIL _____

PERFORMANCE CHECKLIST A.2 PREPARING FOR PHYSICAL ASSESSMENT

	S	U	COMMENTS
1. Gathered appropriate equipment and kept within easy reach during assessment.			
2. Washed hands before and after assessment.			
3. Demonstrated knowledge of body structure and function.			
4. Promoted client comfort and privacy throughout assessment.			
5. Utilized a systematic approach using the 4 basic maneuvers.			
6. Used good lighting and adequate exposure for inspection.			
7. Performed the techniques of palpation and percussion correctly.			
8. Auscultated with stethoscope which has a bell, diaphragm, proper fitting earpieces, and proper length tubing.			
9. Instructed client appropriately throughout assessment.			
10. Conducted assessment in nonthreatening manner.			
11. Conducted assessment from client's right side.			

Additional Comments:

_____

_____

_____

_____

_____

_____

_____

_____

_____

_____

Name _____

Date _____

Instructor _____

Specific Skill Performed _____

Attempt Number _____

PASS _____   FAIL _____

PERFORMANCE CHECKLIST A.3   ASSESSING GENERAL APPEARANCE

	S	U	COMMENTS
1. Assessed client's age.			
2. Noted client's race and sex.			
3. Observed client's body build and posture.			
4. Determined smoothness and coordination of walk.			
5. Observed client's general appearance and nutrition status.			
6. Compared assessment findings to normal characteristics.			
7. Accurately documented description of client's general appearance.			

Additional Comments:

_____

_____

_____

_____

_____

_____

_____

_____

_____

_____

_____

_____

Name _____   Specific Skill Performed _____
Date _____   Attempt Number _____
Instructor _____   PASS _____   FAIL _____

PERFORMANCE CHECKLIST A.4 ASSESSING MENTAL STATUS AND SPEECH

	S	U	COMMENTS
1. Noted client's grooming, type of dress, and hygiene.			
2. Considered lifestyle, culture, age, and socioeconomic group when interpreting results of assessment.			
3. Assessed client's judgment by asking simple questions.			
4. Asked client to interpret proverbs to assess abstract thinking.			
5. Assessed orientation to person, place, and time.			
6. Tested immediate, recent, and remote memory correctly.			
7. Observed client for emotional response or affect.			
8. Assessed level of consciousness. If altered, evaluated whether client is demonstrating obtundation, stupor, or coma.			
9. Noted characteristics of client's speech.			
10. Accurately documented mental status and speech.			

Additional Comments:

_____

_____

_____

_____

_____

_____

_____

_____

_____

_____

_____

Name _____   Specific Skill Performed _____
Date _____   Attempt Number _____
Instructor _____   PASS _____   FAIL _____

PERFORMANCE CHECKLIST A.5 ASSESSING THE SKIN

	S	U	COMMENTS
1. Obtained good light source.			
2. Compared color, temperature, texture, mobility, lesions and vascularity in symmetric body parts.			
3. Inspected skin for general color especially noting skin on palms, soles, sclera, and nails.			
4. Palpated skin for changes in temperature using the dorsum of the hand.			
5. Palpated skin for moisture.			
6. Palpated skin to assess texture. Noted irregularities.			
7. Pinched skin up in appropriate areas and released it to assess turgor.			
8. Observed for skin lesions. Noted size, location, distribution, pattern, color, and type.			
9. If skin lesions present, palpated to assess mobility, contour, and consistency. Applied sterile gloves to palpate draining lesions.			
10. Noted blood circulation of skin and appearance of superficial blood vessels.			
11. Noted location and appearance of edematous areas.			
12. Palpated edematous areas for mobility, consistency, and tenderness.			
13. Pressed finger into edematous area to test for pitting.			
14. Used tape measure to measure edema in one body part compared to symmetrical body part.			
15. Compared assessment findings with normal characteristics.			
16. Documented assessment results correctly and accurately.			

Additional Comments:

_____

_____

Name _____   Specific Skill Performed _____
Date _____   Attempt Number _____
Instructor _____   PASS _____   FAIL _____

PERFORMANCE CHECKLIST A.6   ASSESSING THE HAIR AND SCALP

	S	U	COMMENTS
1. Asked client if any changes in hair or scalp have been noted.			
2. Inspected hair for quality, quantity, and distribution.			
3. Assessed for sudden changes in hair color.			
4. Observed for abnormal facial hair.			
5. Separated hair to take thorough look at scalp.			
6. Used rotary motion with pads of fingers to palpate scalp and skull.			
7. Palpated entire skull beginning with frontal region, then temporal and parietal region to the occipital region.			
8. Compared assessment findings with normal characteristics.			
9. Documented assessment findings correctly and accurately.			

Additional Comments:

_____

_____

_____

_____

_____

_____

_____

_____

_____

_____

_____

_____

Name _____   Specific Skill Performed _____
Date _____   Attempt Number _____
Instructor _____   PASS _____   FAIL _____

PERFORMANCE CHECKLIST A.7   ASSESSING THE FACE AND CRANIAL NERVES

	S	U	COMMENTS
1. Inspected face for size, symmetry, shape, and tics or abnormal movements.			
2. Correctly tested motor and sensory function in the face or the trigeminal nerve.			
3. Correctly tested motor and sensory function of the facial nerve.			
4. Compared assessment findings to normal characteristics.			
5. Documented assessment results accurately and correctly.			

Additional Comments:

_____

_____

_____

_____

_____

_____

_____

_____

_____

_____

_____

_____

_____

_____

Name _____   Specific Skill Performed _____
Date _____   Attempt Number _____
Instructor _____   PASS _____   FAIL _____

PERFORMANCE CHECKLIST A.8   ASSESSING THE EYES

	S	U	COMMENTS
1. Inspected eyes for position and alignment.			
2. Inspected quantity and distribution of eyebrows.			
3. Inspected eyelids for symmetry, position in relation to eyeballs, inflammation, lesions, edema, and ptosis.			
4. Noted excessive dryness or tearing of eye.			
5. Palpated lacrimal sac and observed for expression of fluid.			
6. Inspected conjunctiva and sclera correctly.			
7. Inspected pupils for quality, size, and shape.			
8. Correctly tested pupillary reaction to light and accommodation or oculomotor, trochlear, and abducens nerves.			
9. Performed cardinal positions test correctly.			
10. Performed cover-uncover test correctly.			
11. Performed corneal light reflex test correctly.			
12. Tested optic nerve correctly by assessing visual fields and visual acuity.			
13. Used proper technique to perform ophthalmoscopic examination.			
14. Compared assessment findings to normal characteristics.			
15. Documented assessment correctly and accurately.			

Additional Comments:

_____

_____

_____

_____

_____

_____

Name _____   Specific Skill Performed _____

Date _____   Attempt Number _____

Instructor _____   PASS _____   FAIL _____

PERFORMANCE CHECKLIST A.9 ASSESSING THE EARS

	S	U	COMMENTS
1. Inspected the auricle for color, size, configuration, location, and angle of attachment.			
2. Inspected external ear canal for intactness, general hygiene, a build up of cerumen, discharge, redness, and swelling.			
3. Palpated external ear and mastoid process for nodules and tenderness.			
4. Used proper technique and positioning for otoscopic examination of internal ear canal and eardrum.			
5. Assessed internal ear canal for impacted cerumen, foreign bodies, discharge, masses, redness, and swelling.			
6. Noted landmarks on eardrum and observed for perforations, distorted or absent cone of light, abnormal color, bulging or retraction, discharge, fluid or air bubbles.			
7. Correctly tested the acoustic nerve through auditory acuity, Weber lateralization test, and Rinne air and bone conduction test.			
8. Compared assessment findings to normal characteristics.			
9. Documented assessment findings accurately and correctly.			

Additional Comments:

_____

_____

_____

_____

_____

_____

_____

_____

_____

PERFORMANCE CHECKLIST A.10 **ASSESSING THE NOSE AND SINUSES**

	S	U	COMMENTS
1. Inspected external surface of nose for symmetry in color, size, and shape.			
2. Inspected external septum for symmetry and signs of deviation.			
3. Palpated external nares for tenderness.			
4. Assessed patency of nares correctly.			
5. Used penlight and instructed client to tilt head back to inspect nasal mucosa.			
6. Inspected nasal mucosa for color, moisture, swelling, lesions, or dryness.			
7. Inspected middle and inferior turbinate for color and swelling.			
8. Palpated frontal and maxillary sinuses correctly for tenderness, swelling, thickening, or secretions.			
9. Assessed olfactory nerve function by correctly testing smell.			
10. Compared assessment findings to normal characteristics.			
11. Documented assessment results correctly and accurately.			

Additional Comments:

_____

_____

_____

_____

_____

_____

_____

_____

Name _____

Date _____

Instructor _____

Specific Skill Performed _____

Attempt Number _____

PASS _____   FAIL _____

PERFORMANCE CHECKLIST A.11 ASSESSING THE MOUTH AND PHARYNX

	S	U	COMMENTS
1. Inspected lips for symmetry, color, edema, or surface abnormalities.			
2. Applied gloves.			
3. Palpated lips for moistness, induration, intactness, and lesions.			
4. Pulled down on lower lip, then up on upper lip to inspect gums for color, lesions, inflammation, and bleeding.			
5. Palpated gums for retraction, lesions, swelling, and hypertrophy. Removed dentures if necessary.			
6. Inspected teeth for color, decay, plaque, or missing teeth.			
7. Used tongue blade and penlight to inspect buccal mucosa for color, pigmentation, ulcers, white patches, and nodules.			
8. Inspected and palpated tongue correctly noting symmetry, color, movement, or presence of masses.			
9. Correctly tested function of hypoglossal nerve by observing position and movement of tongue.			
10. Inspected the hard and soft palate for color, lesions, and symmetry.			
11. Correctly tested the glossopharyngeal nerve and the vagus nerve.			
12. Compared assessment findings to normal characteristics.			
13. Documented assessment results accurately and correctly.			

Additional Comments:

_____

_____

_____

_____

_____

_____

Name _____   Specific Skill Performed _____
Date _____   Attempt Number _____
Instructor _____   PASS _____   FAIL _____

PERFORMANCE CHECKLIST A.12 ASSESSING THE NECK

	S	U	COMMENTS
1. Placed client in upright position.			
2. Inspected neck for color, symmetry, masses, enlarged thyroid, enlarged lymph nodes, abnormal pulsations, lesions, and scars.			
3. Palpated neck for changes in temperature and texture.			
4. Instructed client to move neck through entire range of motion.			
5. Used pads of first 2 fingers to palpate lymph nodes correctly and systematically in all appropriate areas.			
6. Palpated thyroid gland correctly for size, shape, symmetry, and the presence of masses.			
7. Correctly palpated the trachea for deviation from midline.			
8. Palpated 1 carotid artery at a time to assess for symmetry, amplitude and rate and rhythm of pulsations.			
9. Auscultated carotid arteries using the bell of the stethoscope to assess for bruits.			
10. Assessed the spinal accessory nerve correctly.			
11. Observed for abnormal or unusual distention in the jugular veins.			
12. Compared assessment findings to normal characteristics.			
13. Documented assessment results accurately and correctly.			

Additional Comments:

_____

_____

_____

_____

_____

_____

_____

Name _____   Specific Skill Performed _____
Date _____   Attempt Number _____
Instructor _____   PASS _____   FAIL _____

PERFORMANCE CHECKLIST A.13 ASSESSING THE CHEST AND LUNGS

	S	U	COMMENTS
1. Identified the reference lines and landmarks on the thorax.			
2. Inspected posterior and anterior chest for the presence of skeletal deformities or abnormalities of the ribs or intercostal spaces.			
3. Assessed rate and rhythm of respirations.			
4. Palpated posterior and anterior chest for tenderness, masses, and sinus tracts.			
5. Assessed respiratory excursion correctly and noted symmetry of chest movement.			
6. Palpated fremitus correctly.			
7. Correctly percussed posterior, anterior, and lateral chest.			
8. Assessed diaphragmatic excursion correctly.			
9. Auscultated thorax using the diaphragm of the stethoscope and comparing 1 side of the thorax to the other.			
10. Auscultated for spoken and whispered sounds.			
11. Compared assessment findings to normal characteristics.			
12. Documented assessment results accurately and correctly.			

Additional Comments:

_____

_____

_____

_____

_____

_____

_____

_____

PERFORMANCE CHECKLIST A.14 **ASSESSING THE HEART**

	S	U	COMMENTS
1. Identified anatomical landmarks on chest.			
2. Inspected precordial points from an angle for abnormal pulsations or lifts. Noted the apical impulse.			
3. Palpated each precordial point correctly for abnormal pulsations, thrills, or lifts.			
4. Palpated apical area along 4th or 5th intercostal space to locate PMI.			
5. Auscultated heart sounds in each precordial area with both the bell and the diaphragm.			
6. Listened to first sound at each precordial area heard best at apex of heart.			
7. Listened to second sound at each precordial area heard best at the base of the heart.			
8. Listened for third heart sound with bell at mitral area.			
9. Listened for fourth heart sound with bell at mitral area.			
10. Listened at each precordial area and in sitting, supine and left lateral positions for all sounds.			
11. Compared assessment findings with normal characteristics.			
12. Document assessment correctly.			

Additional Comments:

_____

_____

_____

_____

_____

_____

_____

Name _____
Date _____
Instructor _____

Specific Skill Performed _____
Attempt Number _____
PASS _____   FAIL _____

PERFORMANCE CHECKLIST A.15 **ASSESSING THE BREASTS**

	S	U	COMMENTS
1. Protected client's privacy.			
2. Instructed client on self-breast examination as you went through assessment.			
3. Inspected breasts for size, symmetry, contour, and appearance of skin in all correct positions.			
4. Inspected the nipples for size, shape, rashes, ulcerations, and discharge.			
5. Carefully lifted breasts to inspect underneath.			
6. Correctly palpated supraclavicular, infraclavicular, and axillary lymph nodes with client in sitting position. Noted consistency, mobility, and tenderness.			
7. Palpated breasts with client in supine position and pillow under scapula on side to be palpated.			
8. Instructed client to raise arm above head on side to be palpated.			
9. Gently used finger pads in a rotating movement in all 4 quadrants of both breasts including areolae, tails of breasts and axillae.			
10. Maintained continuous finger contact with tissue during palpation.			
11. Compressed the areola and nipple of each breast to check for discharge.			
12. Compared assessment findings to normal characteristics.			
13. Documented findings correctly and accurately describing the breast in 4 quadrants or as on the face of a clock.			

Additional Comments:

_____

_____

_____

_____

Name _____   Specific Skill Performed _____

Date _____   Attempt Number _____

Instructor _____   PASS _____   FAIL _____

PERFORMANCE CHECKLIST A.16 ASSESSING THE ABDOMEN

	S	U	COMMENTS
1. Asked client to empty bladder prior to assessing abdomen.			
2. Placed client in supine position with arms at sides and knees slightly flexed.			
3. Protected client's privacy while exposing entire abdomen.			
4. Identified system of landmarks for mapping abdominal regions such as 4 quadrants or 9 sections.			
5. Inspected by looking across abdominal surface for contour, symmetry, skin, umbilicus, peristalsis, and pulsations.			
6. Auscultated with diaphragm of stethoscope in each quadrant or section of abdomen.			
7. Auscultated using the bell of the stethoscope for bruits in all correct areas.			
8. Percussed in all quadrants or sections of the abdomen leaving any painful areas for last. Identified liver borders and spleen.			
9. Palprated in all quadrants or sections of abdomen for tenderness, muscle tone, stiffening and masses, using palmer surfaces of fingertips for light palpation, then placing one hand on top of the other for deep palpation.			
10. Palpated liver correctly with fingertips below lower border of liver dullness.			
11. Palpated spleen correctly and attempted to palpate kidneys correctly .			
12. Used fintertips to palpate aorta in epgastric area.			
13. Elicited abdominal reflex.			
14. Compared assessment findings with normal characteristics.			
15. Documented assessment findings correctly and accurately according to quadrants or sections.			

PERFORMANCE CHECKLIST A.17 PREPARING TO EXAMINE THE GENITALS AND RECTUM

	S	U	COMMENTS
1. Explained actions to client beforehand.			
2. Avoided sexually provocative actions or statements.			
3. Performed examination wearing gloves.			
4. Used firm touch.			
5. Provided for client privacy.			
6. Performed examination as quickly and efficiently as possible.			
7. Warmed instruments and used lubricant to minimize discomfort.			
8. Maintained professional attitude.			

Additional Comments:

_____

_____

_____

_____

_____

_____

_____

_____

_____

_____

_____

_____

_____

Name _____   Specific Skill Performed _____
Date _____   Attempt Number _____
Instructor _____   PASS _____   FAIL _____

PERFORMANCE CHECKLIST A.18 ASSESSING THE MALE GENITALIA

	S	U	COMMENTS
1. Inspected structures of penis for lesions, odor, discharge or inflammation.			
2. Inspected anterior and posterior scrotal skin for sores, rashes, swelling, lumps, or veins.			
3. Asked client to cough while observing for groin masses and bulging.			
4. Palpated penis for tenderness or induration.			
5. Palpated testes and epididymis of scrotum for size, shape, consistency, and tenderness or nodules.			
6. Instructed client on self-testicular exam.			
7. Palpated inguinal ring and canal correctly.			
8. Compared assessment findings to normal characteristics.			
9. Documented assessment findings accurately and correctly.			

Additional Comments:

_____

_____

_____

_____

_____

_____

_____

_____

_____

_____

_____

PERFORMANCE CHECKLIST A.19 ASSESSING THE FEMALE GENITALIA

	S	U	COMMENTS
1. Instructed client to empty bladder prior to examination.			
2. Gathered appropriate equipment and placed within easy reach.			
3. Placed client in lithotomy position.			
4. Touched client's thigh prior to contact with the genitalia.			
5. Inspected external genitalia for inflammation, discharge, ulceration or nodules.			
6. Noted character and distribution of pubic hair.			
7. Inspected and palpated Bartholin's glands correctly.			
8. Inserted lubricated, gloved index finger into vagina and located cervix.			
9. Instructed client to strain down while observing for bulging of vaginal walls.			
10. Chose the correct size speculum. Warmed and lubricated with water before inserting.			
11. Depressed perineum using first 2 fingers of nondominant hand.			
12. Using dominant hand, introduced speculum obliquely into the vagina.			
13. Inserted speculum at 45° angle against rectal wall.			
14. When speculum completely inserted, rotated it to transverse position and opened it slowly to visualize cervix.			
15. Tighten set screw to keep speculum open.			
16. Inspected cervix for color, position, and surface characteristics.			
17. Correctly obtained an endocervical swab, if appropriate, using cotton-tipped applicator. Smeared gently on glass slide and sprayed with fixative.			
18. Correctly obtained cervical scrape using wooden spatula. Placed specimen on glass slide and prepared slide correctly.			

	S	U	COMMENTS
19. Inspected vaginal mucosa for color, inflammation, ulceration, or masses as speculum is withdrawn.			
20. Closed speculum blades completely before withdrawing speculum.			
21. Lubricated gloved index and middle fingers.			
22. Palpated perineum for tenderness and nodules.			
23. Placed fingers into vagina and palpated cervix for position, size, mobility, and tenderness.			
24. Placed other hand on abdomen slightly above symphysis pubis.			
25. Correctly palpated size, shape, consistency and mobility of uterus.			
26. Palpated adnexa correctly. Noted size, shape, consistency, mobility, and tenderness.			
27. Compared assessment findings to normal characteristics.			
28. Documented assessment results correctly and accurately.			

Additional Comments:

_____

_____

_____

_____

_____

_____

_____

_____

_____

_____

_____

_____

_____

PERFORMANCE CHECKLIST A.20 ASSESSING THE RECTUM

	S	U	COMMENTS
1. Inspected anal area by gently spreading the buttocks. Noted hemorrhoids, rashes, inflammation, and ulcers.			
2. Applied gloves and lubricated finger.			
3. Applied gentle pressure at lower edge of rectum with index finger.			
4. Instructed client to strain down or to take a deep breath as you inserted your index finger into the anal canal.			
5. Assessed sphincter tone.			
6. Rotated finger to palpate all walls of the rectum for polyps, irregularities or tenderness.			
7. Examined prostate noting size, shape, nodules, consistency, and tenderness.			
8. Gently withdrew finger from rectum.			
9. Examined stool on glove for blood or pus.			
10. Gave client tissues to wipe anal area.			
11. Compared assessment findings to normal characteristics.			
12. Documented assessment results correctly and accurately.			

Additional Comments:

_____

_____

_____

_____

_____

_____

_____

_____

Name _____   Specific Skill Performed _____
Date _____   Attempt Number _____
Instructor _____   PASS _____   FAIL _____

PERFORMANCE CHECKLIST A.21 ASSESSING THE UPPER EXTREMITIES

	S	U	COMMENTS
1. Inspected upper extremities beginning at fingertips and moving to shoulders.			
2. Observed skin and nailbeds for symmetry, color, texture, venous pattern, edema, and nail angle.			
3. Palpated brachial, radial and ulnar pulses bilaterally.			
4. Auscultated brachial, radial and ulnar arteries for bruits using the bell of the stethoscope.			
5. Assessed biceps, triceps, and brachioradialis reflexes correctly.			
6. Compared assessment findings to normal characteristics.			
7. Documented assessment results correctly and accurately.			

Additional Comments:

_____

_____

_____

_____

_____

_____

_____

_____

_____

_____

_____

_____

_____

Name _____   Specific Skill Performed _____

Date _____   Attempt Number _____

Instructor _____   PASS _____   FAIL _____

PERFORMANCE CHECKLIST A.22 ASSESSING THE LOWER EXTREMITIES

	S	U	COMMENTS
1. Inspected lower extremities beginning at groin and buttocks and moving to toes.			
2. Observed skin and nailbeds for size, symmetry, venous pattern, color, texture, rashes, ulcers, edema, and hair growth.			
3. Palpated inguinal lymph nodes.			
4. Palpated femoral, popliteal, dorsalis pedis, and posterior tibial pulses bilaterally.			
5. Assessed Homan's sign correctly.			
6. Assessed patellar, ankle, and plantar reflexes correctly.			
7. Compared assessment findings to normal characteristics.			
8. Documented assessment results correctly and accurately.			

Additional Comments:

_____

_____

_____

_____

_____

_____

_____

_____

_____

_____

_____

_____

_____

Name _____   Specific Skill Performed _____
Date _____   Attempt Number _____
Instructor _____   PASS ____   FAIL ____

PERFORMANCE CHECKLIST A.23 ASSESSING THE MOTOR SYSTEM

	S	U	COMMENTS
1. Inspected the voluntary muscles for atrophy, twitching, and involuntary position.			
2. Instructed client to walk across the room to assess gait.			
3. Assessed the client walking a straight line, heel-to-toe.			
4. Correctly assessed Romberg test.			
5. Tested muscle strength of all major muscle groups.			
6. Correctly assessed coordination.			
7. Compared assessment findings to normal characteristics.			
8. Documented assessment results correctly and accurately.			

Additional Comments:

_____

_____

_____

_____

_____

_____

_____

_____

_____

_____

_____

_____

PERFORMANCE CHECKLIST A.24 ASSESSING THE SENSORY SYSTEM

	S	U	COMMENTS
1. Questioned client about areas of numbness or unusual sensation.			
2. Instructed client to close eyes during testing.			
3. Compared sides of body during exam.			
4. Applied stimuli at random.			
5. Correctly assessed for light touch.			
6. Tested temperature response if pain perception is abnormal.			
7. Assessed vibration sense correctly on interphalangeal joints of finger and great toe.			
8. Correctly tested position sense.			
9. Correctly assessed for stereognosis and graphesthesia.			
10. Correctly tested two-point discrimination, point localization, and extinction.			
11. Compared assessment findings to normal characteristics.			
12. Documented assessment results correctly and accurately.			

Additional Comments:

_____

_____

_____

_____

_____

_____

_____

_____

_____

E CHECKLIST A.25 CONCLUDING THE PHYSICAL ASSESSMENT

		S	U	COMMENTS
1.	Helped client to remove lubricant and body secretions from perineal and rectal areas.			
2.	Removed drape and helped client with clothing.			
3.	Disposed of linens and equipment appropriately.			
4.	Discussed findings with client if appropriate.			
5.	Documented all aspects of the assessment accurately and correctly.			

Additional Comments:

_____

_____

_____

_____

_____

_____

_____

_____

_____

_____

_____

_____

_____

_____

_____

_____